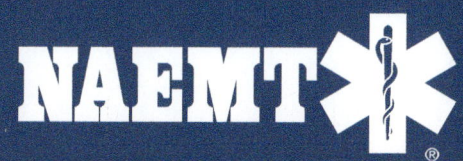

NAEMT

THIRD EDITION

EMS Safety

COURSE MANUAL

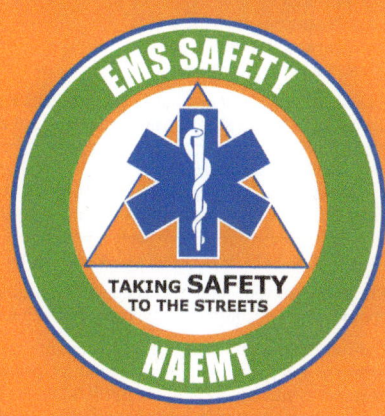

EMS SAFETY
TAKING SAFETY TO THE STREETS
NAEMT

W0113353

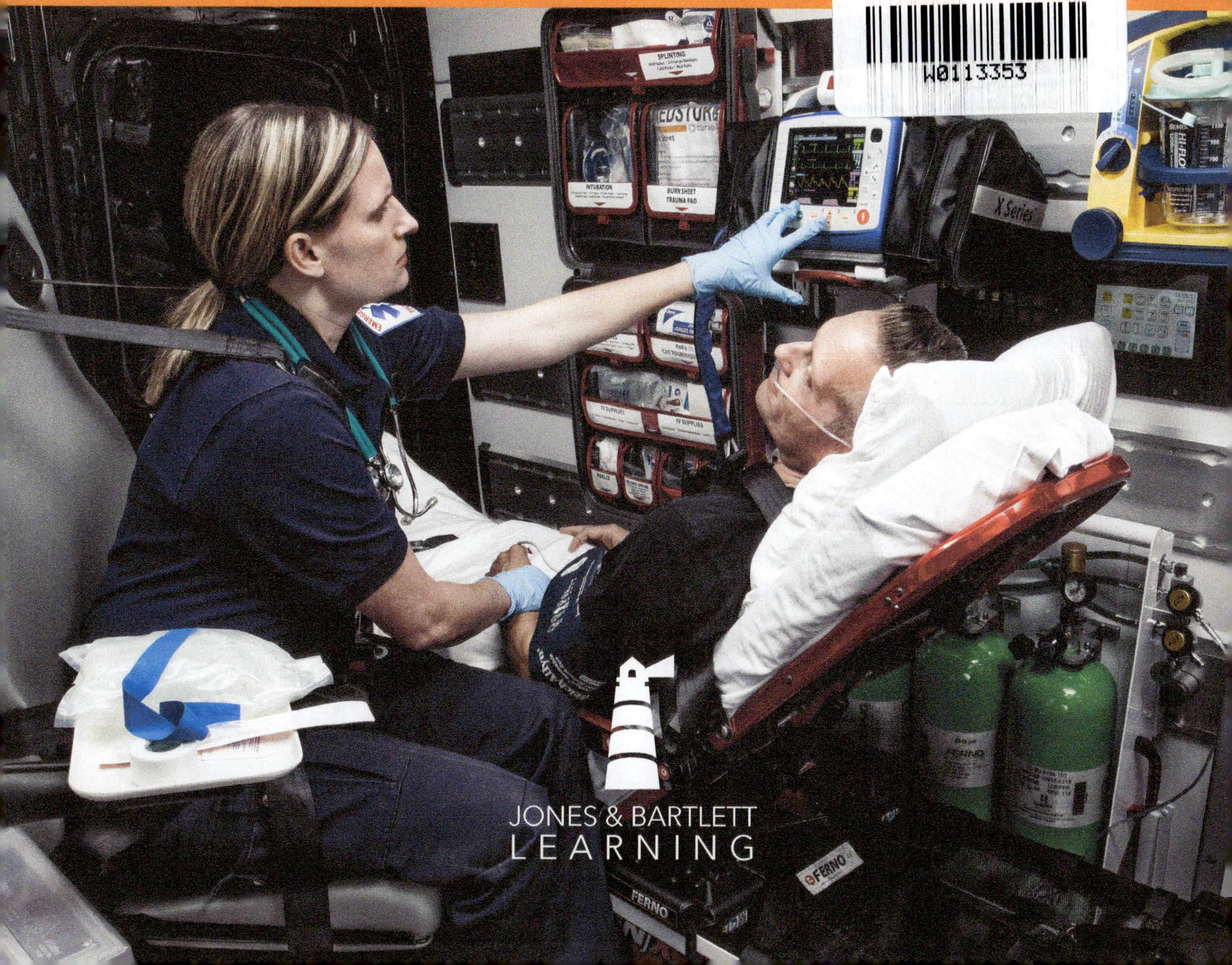

JONES & BARTLETT LEARNING

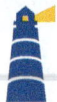

World Headquarters
Jones & Bartlett Learning
25 Mall Road
Burlington, MA 01803
978-443-5000
info@jblearning.com
www.jblearning.com
www.psglearning.com

Jones & Bartlett Learning books and products are available through most bookstores and online booksellers. To contact the Jones & Bartlett Learning Public Safety Group directly, call 800-832-0034, fax 978-443-8000, or visit our website, www.psglearning.com.

Production Credits
Vice President, Product Management: Marisa R. Urbano
Vice President, Content Strategy and Product Implementation:
  Christine Emerton
Director, Product Management: Laura Carney
Director, Content Management: Donna Gridley
Content Strategist: Ashley Procum
Content Strategist: Alexander Belloli
Director, Project Management and Content Services: Karen Scott
Project Manager: Kristen Rogers
Project Specialist: Madelene Nieman
Digital Project Specialist: Angela Dooley
Director of Marketing: Brian Rooney

Vice President, International Sales, Public Safety Group: Matthew Maniscalco
Director, Sales, Public Safety Group: Brian Hendrickson
Content Services Manager: Colleen Lamy
Vice President, Manufacturing and Inventory Control: Therese Connell
Composition: S4Carlisle Publishing Services
Cover & Text Design Design: Scott Moden
Senior Media Development Editor: Troy Liston
Rights & Permissions Manager: John Rusk
Rights Specialist: Liz Kincaid
Cover Image (Title Page): Courtesy of Ferno Washington, Inc.
Printing and Binding: LSC Communications

Library of Congress Cataloging-in-Publication Data
Names: National Association of Emergency Medical Technicians (U.S.) editor.
Title: EMS safety course manual / edited by National Association of
  Emergency Medical Technicians (NAEMT).
Other titles: EMS safety.
Description: Third edition. | Burlington, MA : Jones & Bartlett Learning,
  [2023] | Preceded by EMS safety / EMS Safety Committee of the National
  Association of Emergency Medical Technicians. Second edition. 2017. |
  Includes bibliographical references and index.
Identifiers: LCCN 2021056360 | ISBN 9781284261462 (paperback)
Subjects: MESH: Emergency Medical Technicians | Occupational
  Injuries--prevention & control | Emergency Treatment | Emergency Medical
  Services | Safety Management | United States
Classification: LCC RA975.5.E5 | NLM WA 487.5.E6 | DDC
  362.18--dc23/eng/20220112
LC record available at https://lccn.loc.gov/2021056360

6048

Printed in the United States of America
26 25 24   10 9 8 7 6 5 4 3 2

Brief Contents

Contents

Acknowledgments

EMS Safety Course Manual, Third Edition

EMS Safety Third Edition Author Team

Garrett Hedeen, MHA, NRP
EMS Manager
IU Health Lifeline
Bloomington, Indiana

Michael Kaduce, MPS, NRP
EMT Program Director
UCLA Center for Prehospital Care
Los Angeles, California

Justin Koper, MS, CSP, MTSP-C, FP-C, DICO-C
Continuous Improvement Manager
HealthNet Aeromedical Services
Charleston, West Virginia

Ryan Ockey, BS, NRP
EMS Program Faculty
UCLA Center for Prehospital Care
Los Angeles, California

Jeffrey A. White, MS, CHSP, MTSP-C, FP-C
Director of Safety
HealthNet Aeromedical Services
Charleston, West Virginia

EMS Safety Course Manual, Third Edition Medical Director

Douglas F. Kupas, MD, EMT-P, FAEMS, FACEP
Medical Director, Geisinger EMS
EMS Medical Director, State of Pennsylvania
Director, Resuscitation Program, Geisinger Medical Center
Danville, Pennsylvania

Editorial Consultant to NAEMT for EMS Safety Course Manual, Third Edition

Bob Elling, MPA, Paramedic (retired)
Career Paramedic, Educator, Author, and EMS Advocate
CEO High Quality Endeavors, Ltd.
Hernando, Florida

National Association of Emergency Medical Technicians 2021 Board of Directors

Officers

President: Bruce Evans
President-Elect: Susan Bailey
Immediate Past President: Matt Zavadsky
Secretary: Troy Tuke
Treasurer: Chris Way
Medical Director: Douglas F. Kupas, MD

Directors

Robert Luckritz
Bryan Nelson
Melissa McNally
William Tatum
Eric Van Dusen
Debra Von Seggern-Johnson
Karen Larsen
Macara Trusty
Allison G.S. Knox
Garrett Hedeen

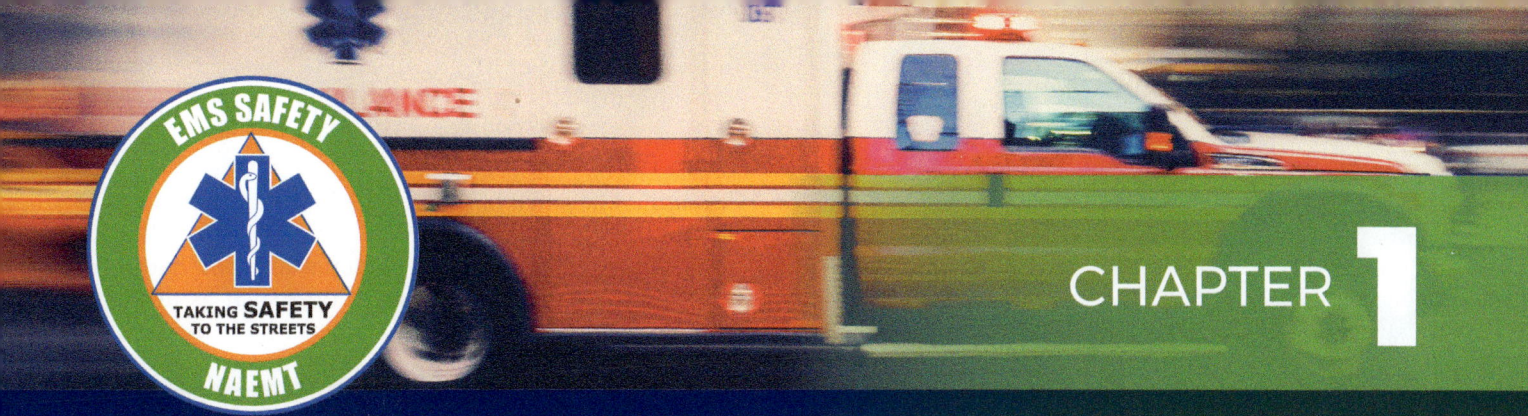

CHAPTER 1

How Safety Impacts Patients and Practitioners

LESSON OBJECTIVES

- Discuss the goals of the EMS Safety course.
- Review EMS practitioner injury and mortality rates.
- Identify best communication and documentation practices.
- Discuss issues of patient safety in EMS.

Scenario

On your way into work, you notice that traffic is becoming congested, and you realize you are going to be late. As you pull into the station, you see that your partner also is just pulling in. You are both 15 minutes late. Both of you quickly grab your gear and toss it in the ambulance as the tones go off. There has been no time to check your ambulance, nor receive a hand-off report from the previous crew.

Dispatch reports that a 61-year-old man is in cardiac arrest. On arrival, your partner opens the side cabinet to retrieve the cardiac monitor and realizes it is not there. You look in the back of the unit and notice that your first-in bag is missing the intubation equipment.

1. How could this situation have been mitigated from the start?
2. What is your first priority in this situation?
3. What actions are required next?

Introduction

Emergency medical services (EMS) is a profession of extremes. One moment, we are dealing with patient care situations that stress our cognitive and psychomotor skills in potentially life-threatening environments. In the next moment, we are performing a routine patient transport. We leap from emotionally charged scenes to emotionally neutral ones, often without the opportunity for physical or mental recovery (**FIGURE 1-1**). The transition from an intense situation to a calm one can be exhausting, and this can lead us to let down our guard during the moments of calm. For example, after running "hot" during a call,

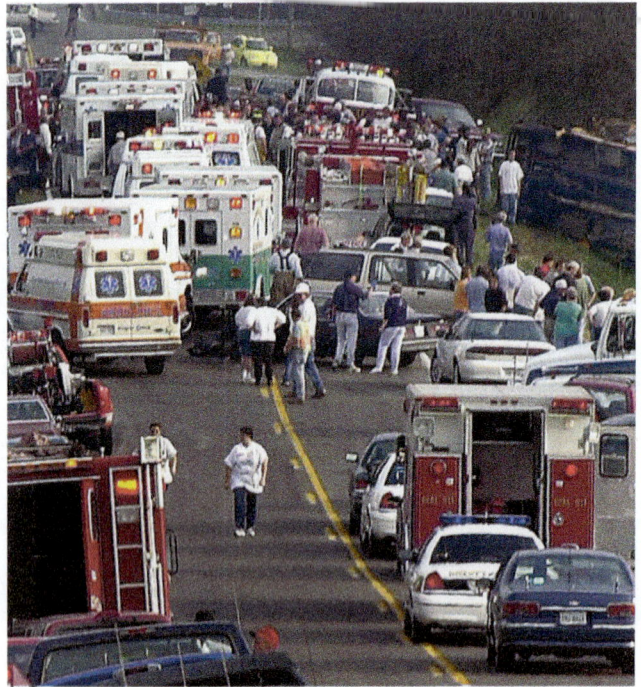

A

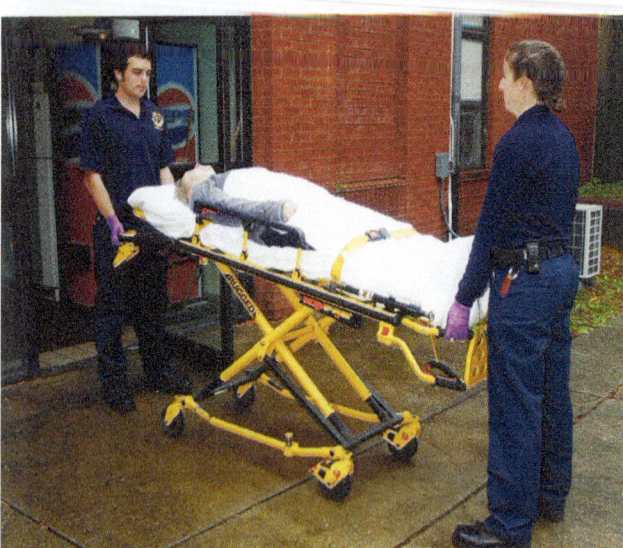

B

FIGURE 1-1 EMS is a profession of extremes. **A.** One moment, you may be dealing with a life-threatening situation. **B.** The next moment, you may be moving a patient.

A. © David Crigger, Bristol Herald Courier/AP Photo; B. © Jones & Bartlett Learning.

we may be less attentive to traffic while driving back to the station after a call.

The constant cycle of crisis and calm may lead us to pay less attention to our surroundings and subsequently fail to process sensorimotor cues in the environment. **Sensorimotor cues** are the sights, sounds, and smells that create an awareness of environmental conditions; this awareness may prompt a behavioral response. For example, the smell of smoke could prompt you to look for a fire.

EMS practitioners and patients are not harmed only in overtly dangerous situations, such as driving in an ice storm. A growing number of patients are injured, sometimes critically, in nonemergent patient-handling events, such as moving a patient from a bed to a stretcher. When a task seems "routine," there is a risk of the mind slipping into **complacency**, which occurs when you believe you are so good at your job that you stop thinking about how to do it properly. When you stop thinking about your job, you lose the ability to maintain situational awareness.

You may be thinking that you have taken driving courses and patient safety training and have participated in a variety of other safety-oriented activities. You have onboard monitoring equipment and powered cots. You use all the appropriate personal protective equipment (PPE) on every call. You know the dangers of intersections, the use of lights and siren, and the plague of distracted drivers. What else can you possibly do to improve your safety? The *NAEMT EMS Safety* course was developed by a team of EMS safety faculty and subject matter experts. The course will explore the preventive measures that you and your colleagues can take to improve personal, patient, and bystander safety. The course will cover the following topic areas, which have been identified as those most vital to EMS professional safety:

- Crew resource management
- Emergency vehicle safety
- Roadway safety
- Patient safety
- Practitioner safety
- Injury and infection prevention
- Personal health

Overall course learning objectives ensure that the student participating in the course will be able to do the following:

- Identify the hazards faced by EMS practitioners.
- Describe the principles of crew resource management.
- Apply techniques to maintain vehicle safety.
- List and assess areas to improve patient safety.
- Identify strategies to ensure practitioner safety.
- Employ the principles of personal health.

Culture of Safety

The primary goal of EMS Safety is to change the culture of safety in the EMS profession and in each organization. There continues to be a need to change the safety culture in which EMS practitioners serve. An organization's safety culture is the product of everyone's competencies,

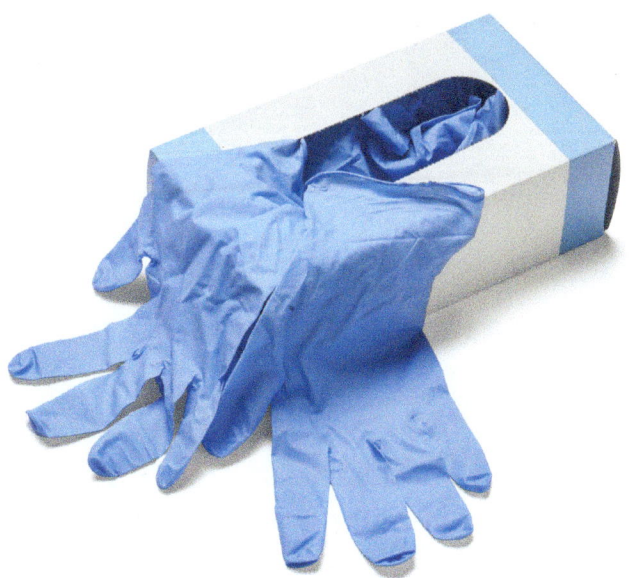

FIGURE 1-2 Safety is in your hands!
© Picsfive/Shutterstock.

4. Evolution of EMS education to include better training on these topics
5. Promulgation of safety standards based on good evidence
6. Incident reporting and investigation

Stay in the Field

Safety is a dynamic issue. Remember the concept of homeostasis from your initial training? Cells constantly engage in a variety of actions to maintain a balanced internal environment. Homeostatic mechanisms work to limit the damage that cells incur when assaulted by everything from hypoxia to mechanical forces. Likewise, EMS practitioners need to develop a set of homeostatic mechanisms—or behaviors— to constantly adapt to the ever-changing environment and limit the potential risks to ourselves, our patients, and bystanders. EMS Safety will teach you how to develop ingrained behaviors that will allow you to adapt naturally to the current situation and address issues before they become threats. Proactive prevention is the key to maintaining your safety and the safety of your partner, patients, and bystanders.

attitudes, and values in determining the commitment to the organization's health and safety programs. EMS Safety is the only national, comprehensive safety course for EMS practitioners. A profession-wide culture of safety is instrumental in creating a safe environment for EMS personnel. The safety of a situation is dynamic and can change at any moment. Weather, traffic flow, and bystanders becoming unruly can all alter scene safety. The decisions that EMS providers make can contribute to creating a culture of safety. The EMS Safety course will provide guidance and introduce behaviors to avoid, prevent, and adapt to safety threats. Everyone, including organizational leaders, EMS practitioners, medical directors, management, and support staff, shares the goal of safety and the continuous improvement required to attain this goal. Leadership and management personnel must share the commitment to a culture of safety, and they should motivate everyone to share the same commitment.

Failure to initiate a culture of safety could have devastating effects. Self-injury prevention is the most valuable service a prehospital practitioner can provide. Safety is in your hands (**FIGURE 1-2**).

The National EMS Culture of Safety project was created in 2009 to improve safety in EMS. The six critical elements to a culture of safety are as follows:

1. Just culture, which encourages reporting of mistakes and near misses, so that errors can be avoided in the future
2. Coordinated support and resources among agencies across the nation
3. A responder and patient safety data system, allowing for better understanding of the scope of some of these issues

The Facts

EMS remains an unsafe profession with a high probability of injury and fatality rate. Whether working for a paid, volunteer, private, fire-based, or government service, all EMS practitioners are at risk. The Centers for Disease Control and Prevention (CDC) reports more than 22,000 EMS personnel are seen in emergency departments for work-related injuries each year. The ways in which injuries occurred based on National Institute for Occupational Safety and Health data from July 2010 to June 2014 are shown in **TABLE 1-1**. The majority of these injuries occurred while responding to an emergency call, which includes patient care and transport. Strains and sprains to the neck and back were the most frequent injuries. Compared with other professions, the following statistics apply to EMS practitioners:

- The fatality rate for EMS practitioners is *2.5 times* the national average.
- The nonfatal injury rate for EMS practitioners is *5 times higher* than for other healthcare workers.
- EMS practitioners are *7 times more likely* than the average worker to miss work as result of injury.

TABLE 1-1 How Did Injuries Occur?	
Injured Workers (per year)	**Causes**
6,000	Body motion (e.g., excessive physical effort, awkward posture, or repetitive movement)
6,000	Exposure to harmful substances (e.g., exposure to blood or respiratory secretions)
4,000	Slips, trips, and falls
2,000	Motor vehicle incidents (e.g., sudden stops, swerves, and crashes)
2,000	Violence/assaults

Reproduced from Centers for Disease Control and Prevention, National Institute for Occupational Safety and Health. Emergency medical services workers: how employers can prevent injuries and exposures [DHHS (NIOSH) Publication No. 2017–194]. Published July 2017. https://www.cdc.gov/niosh/docs/2017-194/pdfs/2017-194 .pdf?id=10.26616/NIOSHPUB2017194

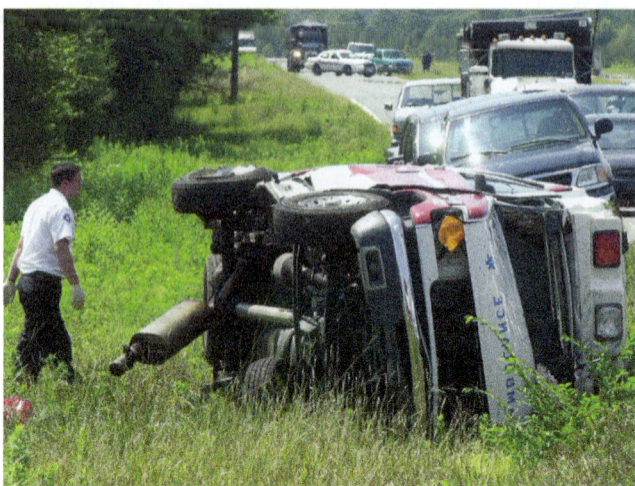

FIGURE 1-3 According to the NHTSA, between 1992 and 2011, there was an average of about 12 motor vehicle crashes involving ambulances per day.

© Gary Lloyd/The Decatur Daily/AP Photo.

Aside from the pain and suffering, the National Safety Council estimates a financial impact of approximately $886.4 billion in 2015 alone from fatal and nonfatal trauma in the United States. The wages and productivity lost was approximately $458 billion. This is more than twice as much as the costs associated with injuries resulting in fatalities.

Motor Vehicle Crashes

According to the National Highway Traffic Safety Administration (NHTSA), between 1992 and 2011, there were 4,500 accidents involving ambulances; this represents an average of about 12 motor vehicle crashes (MVCs) involving ambulances per day (**FIGURE 1-3**). Of those accidents, 65% resulted in property damage, 34% resulted in injuries, and fewer than 1% resulted in fatalities. The breakdown of those fatalities is as follows:

- Ambulance driver: 4%
- Ambulance passenger: 21%
- Occupants of another vehicle: 63%
- Nonoccupants :12%

Of the 34% who were injured, the breakdown is as follows:

- Ambulance driver: 17%
- Ambulance passenger: 29%
- Occupants of another vehicle: 54%

The statistics show that in MVCs involving ambulance crashes, the ambulance driver is less likely to be killed or injured than ambulance passengers, occupants of other vehicles, and nonoccupants. This means that the person responsible for driving the ambulance safely carries the least amount of personal risk in the event of an MVC. The presence of a moving ambulance should not be a hazard to the general public, and the general public should not become "collateral damage" because of an MVC with an ambulance.

In MVCs involving ambulances, 58% of accidents were lights-and-siren events, and 42% were nonemergent driving events. Thus, nonemergent driving events pose an almost equal risk of an MVC as lights-and-siren events. This is one reason it is critical to be aware of potential safety hazards and be proactive about safe driving.

Communications

Maintaining healthy communication with colleagues, bystanders, and patients will assist in creating a safe environment. Always maintain situational awareness and communicate concerns to your partner(s). To practice proactive accident prevention, everyone needs to be aware of the potential hazards. The effectiveness of situational awareness is amplified when EMS practitioners communicate their findings with each other. Be proactive regarding accident prevention by communicating all findings with your team. Situational awareness is a common practice used in law enforcement to ensure the safety of oneself and other peer officers (this topic is discussed further in Chapter 2, *Crew Resource*

Management). EMS personnel should designate one person to maintain contact with the patient while the other person remains alert for scene safety issues.

However, this awareness of safety issues will not occur if interpersonal barriers exist. Interpersonal barriers lead to increased injuries and fatalities. An interpersonal barrier is something preventing clear and open communication among people, such as language barriers, fear of speaking in front of others, or the effects of a stroke. Failing to provide a report to hospital staff of assessment findings or treatment mistakes out of fear of criticism is an example of an interpersonal barrier. EMS practitioners should have a strong desire to protect each other, including from any criticism for speaking up about safety.

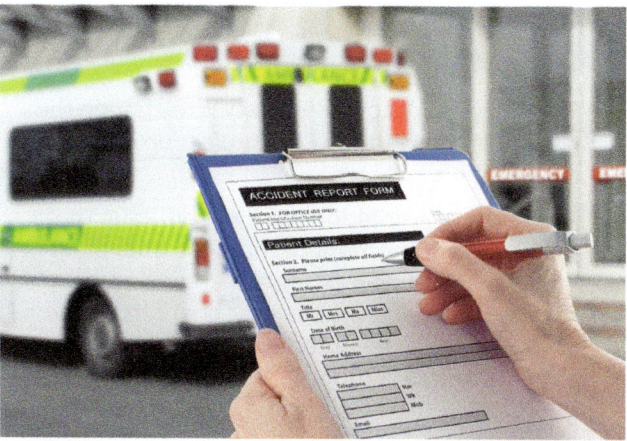

FIGURE 1-4 Documentation is critical.
© Pixsooz/Shutterstock.

In the Field

All healthcare personnel must be aware of safety "red flags" and feel comfortable addressing them. Examples include driving at unsafe speeds, distraction from the roadway, lack of restraints for patient or self, improper lifting techniques, and patient behavior that may lead to an angry outburst or assault. Can you think of others?

Limiting background noise and distractions will improve communication between the healthcare team and the patient. Sometimes this is as simple as turning off the television, or turning down the radio, or asking bystanders to step outside if speaking loudly is disruptive. Always keep your communications equipment with you and listen to your instincts. If the situation does not feel right, leave and call for help.

Documentation

Effective documentation is critical in preventing future safety issues. Documenting all practices, both safe and unsafe, will assist in promoting a culture of safety in an organization. Recognizing and implementing safety awareness can lead to reduced injuries and fatalities in the workplace. Incident/accident reports should be completed as soon as possible after an incident has occurred (**FIGURE 1-4**). Ensure you tell a complete story of the incident occurrence. Effective documentation of the incident, including unsafe practices, could lead to increased awareness of behaviors or policies that can impact injuries and fatalities.

Effective communication and documentation are critical components to implement a culture of safety. There should be no administrative barriers to solving safety issues. EMS leadership should spearhead a culture of safety by instituting an injury prevention policy, maintaining adherence to the policy, and rewarding positive performance. An "open door" policy should be in place for personnel to address safety concerns. People who report a problem should not be identified by coworkers or supervisors as contributing to a problem. The manner in which a problem will be solved and the timeline for the execution of the solution should be shared with everyone in the agency. The inability to completely fix a problem should be shared as well.

Effective documentation is critical to preventing future safety issues. Organizational policy should include the appropriate means to document unsafe practices, and it should be made available to all employees. Providing the flexibility for anonymous reporting of unsafe practices could provide comfort and protection to employees who fear retribution.

CHAPTER WRAP-UP

- The goal of the EMS Safety course is to create a culture of safety in EMS.
- Self-injury prevention is the most valuable service a prehospital practitioner can provide.
- Everyone is responsible for the commitment to fostering a culture of safety.
- Effective communication and documentation are critical components to implementing a culture of safety.

SUMMARY

- The primary goal of EMS Safety is to change the culture of safety in the EMS profession and in each organization.

- The safety of a situation is a dynamic issue that changes from moment to moment. EMS practitioners need to develop a set of ingrained behaviors to constantly adapt to the ever-changing environment and limit the potential risks to ourselves, our patients, and bystanders.

- A profession-wide culture of safety is instrumental in creating a safe environment for EMS personnel.

- EMS is a dangerous job for both professional and volunteer EMS practitioners. The fatality rate for EMS practitioners is 2.5 times the national average. EMS practitioners are 3 times more likely than average workers to miss work as a result of injury.

- Driving carries a significant amount of risk. According to the NHTSA, between 1992 and 2011, an average of about 12 MVCs involving ambulances occurred per day.

- There must be an equal level of awareness and focus given to operating nonemergently and to driving with lights and siren on.

- The National EMS Culture of Safety project was created in 2009 to improve safety in EMS.

- Healthy communication with colleagues, bystanders, and patients will assist in creating a safe environment.

- All healthcare personnel must be aware of safety "red flags" and feel comfortable addressing them.

- Effective documentation is critical to preventing future safety issues.

- EMS practitioners have the right and the responsibility to insist on a safe work environment.

GLOSSARY

complacency A feeling of satisfaction with one's own performance to the point of not recognizing the potential for errors.

sensorimotor cues Sights, sounds, and smells that create an awareness of environmental conditions; this awareness may prompt a behavioral response.

REFERENCES

Centers for Disease Control and Prevention. Emergency Medical Services Workers: How Employers Can Prevent Injuries and Exposures. DHHS (NIOSH) Publication 2017-194. Published July 1, 2017. doi:10.26616/nioshpub2017194

Centers for Disease Control and Prevention. Inside NIOSH: study characterizes injuries and exposures among EMS workers. *Research Rounds*. 2017;3(3). Accessed January 6, 2021. https://www.cdc.gov/niosh/research-rounds/resroundsv3n3.html

De Castro AB. Handle with care: the American Nurses Association campaign to address work-related musculoskeletal disorders. *Online J Issues Nurs*. 2004;9(3):3.

Maguire BJ, Hunting KL, Smith GS, Levick NR. Occupational fatalities in emergency medical services: a hidden crisis. *Ann Emer Med*. 2002;40:625-632.

Maguire BJ, Smith S. Injuries and fatalities among emergency medical technicians in the United States. *Prehosp Disaster Med*. 2013;28(4):376-382. doi:10.1017/s1049023x13003555

National Association of Emergency Medical Technicians. *AMLS: Advanced Medical Life Support: An Assessment-Based Approach*. 3rd ed. Jones & Bartlett Learning; 2021.

National Association of Emergency Medical Technicians. *PHTLS: Prehospital Trauma Life Support*. 9th ed. Jones & Bartlett Learning; 2020.

Page D. Studies show dangers of working in EMS. *JEMS*. Published October 31, 2011. Accessed January 11, 2021. https://www.jems.com/operations/studies-show-dangers-working-ems/

Reichard AA, Marsh SM, Moore PH. Fatal and nonfatal injuries among emergency medical technicians and paramedics. *Prehosp Emerg Care*. 2011;15(4):511-517. doi:10.3109/10903127.2011.598610

Reichard AA, Marsh SM, Tonozzi TR, Konda S, Gormley MA. Occupational injuries and exposures among emergency medical services workers. *Prehosp Emerg Care*. 2017;21(4):420-431. doi:10.1080/10903127.2016.1274350

U.S. Bureau of Labor Statistics. National Census of Fatal Occupational Injuries in 2015; 2016. Accessed January 6, 2021. https://www.bls.gov/news.release/pdf/cfoi.pdf

CHAPTER 2

Crew Resource Management

LESSON OBJECTIVES

- Discuss crew resource management.
- Identify human errors and unsafe actions.
- Model effective communication.
- Demonstrate situational awareness.
- Differentiate leadership and followership responsibilities.

Scenario

You are working the night shift as a field training officer, and your partner is a "newbie." Your unit is dispatched to a patient in respiratory distress. On your arrival at a single-family home, you are directed upstairs where, in the back bedroom, you find a 44-year-old man in severe respiratory distress. The patient is morbidly obese, at over 500 pounds. He is sweating heavily, unable to speak in full sentences, and a quick assessment of his lung sounds shows bilateral crackles.

While you and your partner are having a quick discussion on the best course of treatment and how you are going to move the patient safely to the ambulance, the patient goes into respiratory arrest. You realize there are a dozen things that need to be done immediately, including managing the patient's airway, figuring out how to get him out to the ambulance safely, and dealing with his upset family.

Your partner contacts the dispatcher and requests additional resources. Shortly, a fire engine, two police cars, and another ambulance show up to assist you. An EMS supervisor is en route as well. The fire captain tells you that they are going to bring in a rescue company to move the patient. A member of the ambulance crew argues that the patient should be moved immediately. His partner begins arguing with the patient's mother about which hospital the patient will be transferred to, while the police officers are trying to usher the rest of the family out of the bedroom.

1. What are your primary nonclinical priorities?
2. What is one of the best tools you have at your disposal to manage the scene?
3. How do you deal with conflicting opinions on the best course of treatment?

Introduction

Emergency medical services (EMS) practitioners need to speak up when it comes to safety because poor communication, weak teamwork, and bravado are the top causes of injuries and line-of-duty deaths. So the question is, why don't we, as EMS practitioners, speak up when we see something out of place or have an alternative solution based on previous experience? All too often, EMS has created an environment where the communication path travels in one direction, from the senior authority on down to the trainee. In addition, EMS practitioners may not speak up because of a fear of being wrong, reprisal, and embarrassment. By implementing crew resource management, EMS agencies can ensure that communication paths remain open and that all EMS practitioners at every level of position and experience feel empowered to communicate. The collective goal is safety and for all EMS practitioners to be engaged and responsible for the safety of their partners, their crew, and their patients.

Crew Resource Management

Crew resource management (CRM) is a tool originally instituted by NASA and the airline industry in the 1980s to optimize performance and outcomes by reducing the effect of human error through using all available resources. After the UAL Flight 173 airline crash on December 29, 1978, in a residential area of Portland, Oregon, which killed 10 people, the airline industry developed CRM training for their airline crews (**FIGURE 2-1**). This collision occurred due to

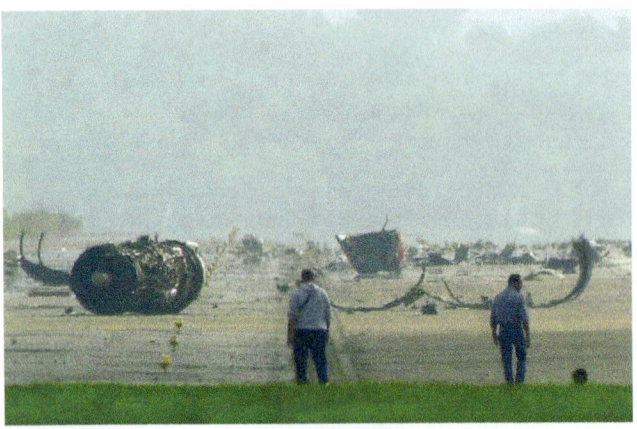

FIGURE 2-1 Crew resource management was instituted by the airline industry in 1980 after the UAL Flight 173 crash to improve collective situational awareness and communication among the airplane's crew.
© Luca Bruno/AP Photo.

human error, and better communications could have prevented it. When the landing gear light failed to illuminate, the pilots delayed landing while working on a solution. In the meantime, they were not monitoring their fuel reserves and they ran out of fuel and crashed!

The goal of CRM training is to enable high-performance teams, such as airline or ambulance crews, to achieve and maintain collective **situational awareness**. Like the airline industry, mistakes in EMS can be fatal, and thus implementing techniques to reduce risk leads to better outcomes. Situational awareness is the state of being aware of what is happening in order to understand how information, events, and a person's actions will affect his or her goals and objectives, both now and in the immediate future. Although we often equate situational awareness to scene safety, CRM applies to all surroundings, including procedures performed while caring for patients. Although the individual is typically the root cause of errors, processes also need to be examined to ensure that tools are in place (i.e., policies, procedures, and information like hardware/software/humanware) to minimize errors and reduce negative consequences.

CRM has been adopted by many **high-reliability organizations (HROs)**, including EMS, fire services, the Coast Guard, and air medical services, to reduce injuries and accidents and improve patient care. HROs are organizations that operate in high-risk environments, such as those associated with law enforcement, fire and EMS, power and utilities, chemical factories, health care, and air traffic control. A common trait among HROs is that their margin for error is minuscule, and the fallout from an adverse event could be disastrous. Critical HRO components include mindfulness, an inclination toward inquiry and doubt as a means of evaluating and updating standard procedures, attention to the complexities of an emergency incident, commitment to resilience, and a willingness to defer to expertise.

Lessons Learned

CRM lessons learned through incident investigation reveal that errors are not random. In fact, they can be predicted based on previous near misses. Even though most errors are unintentional, errors are nonetheless predictable. Although the contributor to the error may not intend harm to anyone, mistakes in the EMS profession can lead to injury to patients or to our partner. Errors arise from poor communication, poor teamwork, and not paying attention. Tracking of near misses and errors can lead to a better understanding of behavior and lead to solutions. In 2017, it was noted that over 251,000 deaths were a direct result of medical error. We could reduce deaths and injuries by mitigating errors.

For example, checklists, a tactic of CRM, are used to ensure all equipment is present in the ambulance and in working order, thus mitigating equipment failure—or missing equipment—as an error.

In the Field

One of the elements the airline industry developed to combat complacency is the checklist. A pilot may have 10,000 hours in the cockpit with zero adverse events, but before every takeoff and every landing, he or she reviews the proper procedures using a checklist that details the steps that must be completed to ensure a successful takeoff, flight, and landing. This is something that EMS practitioners should adopt when performing high-risk or complicated procedures such as rapid sequence intubation (RSI).

Additional checklists are used for key parts of procedures, complex care bundles, looking for high-risk factors in patient refusal, or in the nontransport of stable patients.

Over the last 20 years, fatal accidents in the airline industry have reduced significantly. Two examples with the presence of CRM include UAL Flight 232 and USA Flight 1549. In the UAL Flight 232 crash on July 19, 1989, the hydraulics system failed, leading the pilots to make an emergency landing in Sioux City, Iowa, at the airport. There were 185 survivors and 112 fatalities. Without the skill, experience, and communication between the crew, the number of survivors would have been zero. In the USA Flight 1549 crash on January 15, 2009, Captain Chesley "Sully" Sullenberger landed in the Hudson River following a bird strike. All 155 passengers and crew survived—a prime example of success through using a checklist, team communication, and situational awareness.

Human Error

Incident investigation finds that errors are not random in EMS. People cause accidents by making errors. Errors arise from poor communication, poor teamwork, and not paying attention. EMS practitioners can reduce deaths and injuries by mitigating errors. One of the basic goals of CRM is to reduce errors, because errors are costly to both an EMS agency and EMS practitioners. In the event of a collision, the EMS agency may lose the use of the vehicle or incur the cost of repairs, lawsuits, and workers' compensation claims. If an ambulance crew member is injured, he or she may suffer lost wages or a permanent disability.

In 1990, British psychologist James Reason created the Swiss Cheese Model (SCM) of accident causation to show how accidents occur (**FIGURE 2-2**). The model is a strategy used to address the risks associated with a systems approach to patient safety. Each slice of cheese is viewed as a plan or safeguard, and the holes

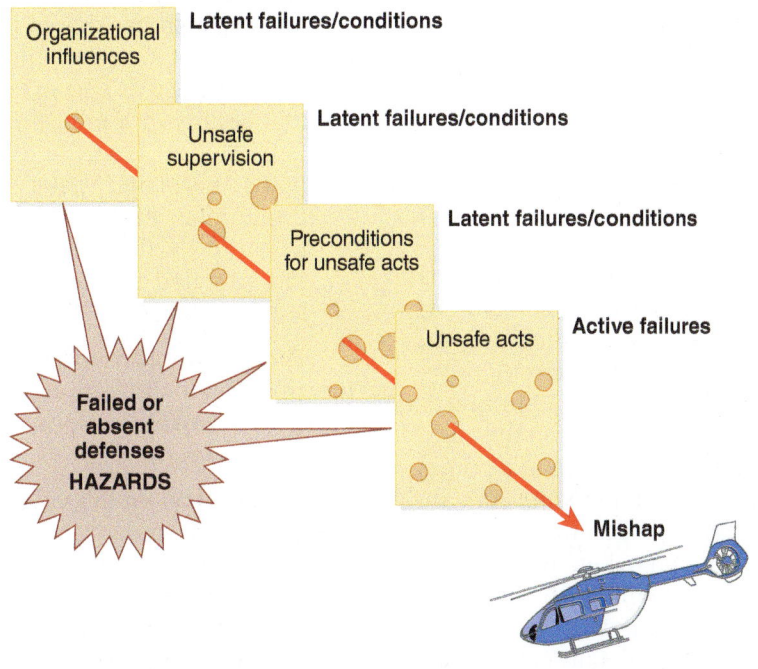

FIGURE 2-2 The Swiss Cheese Model.

Reproduced from Reason J. *Human Error*. Cambridge University Press, Cambridge, UK. 1990.

are examples of hazards or errors that could potentially lead to harm in a patient. Errors could include failing to follow appropriate procedure, individual decision making, or system-wide failures. These layers of "cheese" are staggered and allow an error to get through one hole but be caught by the following mitigation system in place. However, disaster strikes when all the holes align. The use of training, policies, situational awareness, tracking of near misses, checklists, and other recommendations discussed in this chapter will ensure that human error is avoided before a situation ends in patient harm.

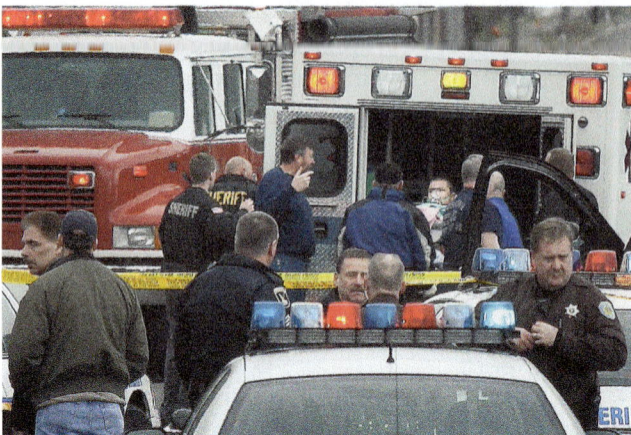

FIGURE 2-3 The chaotic and complex emergencies that EMS practitioners respond to require that they maintain the absolute highest state of alertness and attention at all times.
© Jason Hunt/The Coeur d'Alene Press/AP Photo.

In the Field

James Reason's Swiss Cheese Model includes the following "slices":

- Education
- Training
- Policies
- Technology
- Communication
- Checklists

How do these elements align in your agency? Do you see the potential for an error to slip through the holes?

Situational Awareness

Situational awareness has three primary components: (1) an awareness of the surroundings and how individuals are supposed to interact with the surroundings; (2) the reality of the situation; and (3) individual perceptions of the situation. Situational awareness is an internal active evaluation process that goes on constantly, much like scene size-up. EMS practitioners must update their situational awareness constantly by observing their surroundings, evaluating their options, and communicating with those around them.

The dynamic, fluid emergencies that EMS practitioners respond to require that they maintain the absolute highest state of alertness and attention at all times (**FIGURE 2-3**). Because EMS practitioners are human, loss of situational awareness does occur. This loss of situational awareness is common when EMS practitioners perform routine tasks in familiar surroundings. Later, as EMS practitioners gain experience, they often pay less attention to the mundane details of everyday operations. However, these details can become important as a situation becomes complex.

Maintaining situational awareness is a skill that can be taught. The following essential behaviors help teams maintain situational awareness:

- Asking yourself, "What can go wrong?" This should be a challenging question. What poses the biggest risk? What is the smallest risk? What would happen if either of those things occurred? How would you work with your team to regain control of the situation?
- Reducing the opportunity for unnecessary distraction. On the way to the call, cell phones should be off, and you should be focusing on the information that dispatch has shared (**FIGURE 2-4**).
- Regularly stating the primary mission of the team. Once distracted, a team can head off in a direction that results in a critical loss of situational awareness. This is directly tied to the concept of "Who's flying the plane?" Pilots know that regardless of the number of distractions, their primary mission is still to fly the plane. In a medical context, this can be stated as: "Let's bag the patient. X, A, B, C, let's not forget the basics."

The following are several of the more common factors that lead to distraction or loss of situational awareness. *These* **unsafe actions** *can lead to errors, injuries, death, and destruction!*

- **Ambiguity.** Ambiguity refers to something that can be interpreted in multiple ways. Team members who make ambiguous statements are usually trying to make sense of their surroundings or the situation. They often see something that does not fit, and their statements are designed to express concern without overtly stating that they do not know what is going on. Pay attention to random,

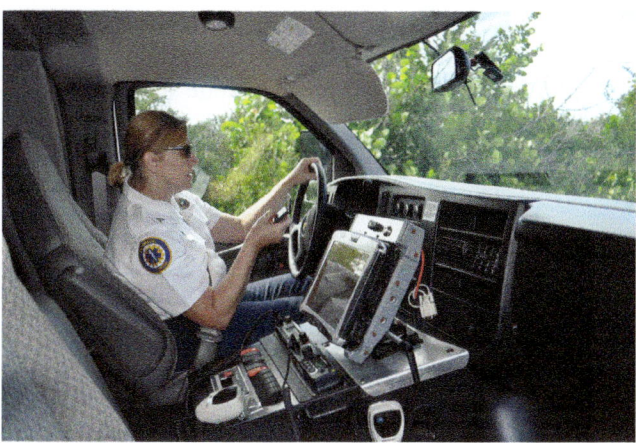

FIGURE 2-4 Emergency vehicle operators should be completely focused on driving, not distractions such as cell phones.

Courtesy of Sunstar Paramedics.

ambiguous statements and "close the loop" by asking for clarification. "What specifically is your concern? What do you see that is bothering you?" These types of questions help provide clarity and understanding. Ambiguous statements can also include inconsistent terminology, which is why it is vital to use plain text instead of slang when speaking (be clear and concise, avoiding jargon and specialized terminology). Ambiguity in situations must also be brought out and clearly stated. For example, if it is not clear who is responsible for picking up the gear at the end of a call, ask, "Would you like me to pack up?" Clear communications will avoid leaving equipment behind on scene. Another example is protocols with different drug dosages (e.g., dosages that are weight based). Medication errors are extremely common in health care. Effective communication to include clarifying drug dosages (e.g., echo back to medical control) with practitioners could prevent errors. If a statement or situation appears ambiguous, work to provide clarity.

- **Fixation.** Fixation is common when there are multiple distractions. In fact, one method humans use to improve performance is to consciously block out things that are not directly tied to their primary objective. On the other hand, a preoccupation or focus on one item, excluding all others, is often referred to as tunnel vision. In EMS, this can take the form of EMS practitioners paying so much attention to one procedure that they ignore other important cues—for example, treating the bleeding from a knife wound but not considering who stabbed the patient and whether the perpetrator is still present on scene. Another example would be

In the Field

Ambiguity can also be a problem when different agencies use different signals, procedures, or terms. Sometimes this can even occur within the same organization. For instance, an EMS practitioner might be asked to "give 10 of Benadryl." Did the sender mean 10 milligrams or 10 milliliters? In most cases, the difference in meaning is significant and needs to be clarified.

The best way to deal with terminology issues is for team members to practice repeating back what they think they heard or what they understand to be correct, not exactly what the person said. "I understand you want 10 milliliters of Benadryl, or 50 milligrams. Is that correct?" For procedural differences, it is best in advance of any incident to collaborate with various agencies to standardize regional practices and procedures, particularly those related to safety.

treating a critical patient involved in a motor vehicle collision on a busy highway and not considering the risk posed by continued traffic.

- **Distraction.** Distraction is something that interferes with concentration or takes your attention away from the task at hand. Dealing with distraction is an skill developed over time. EMS practitioners need to regularly ask about the removal of distracting elements. Will removing certain elements reduce their overall situational awareness or contribute to their ability to concentrate on the most important tasks and objectives? For example, while driving, is the emergency vehicle operator distracted by the radio, mobile data terminal (MDT), cell phones, GPS or electronic mapping systems, conversation with a partner, or his or her emotions? Or are they distracted by nontangible things like coworker disputes, financial concerns, and relationship concerns? Failure to handle a distraction effectively could lead to errors. A simple action such as cutting down on excess noise and nonessential conversation (implementing a sterile cockpit) could improve your overall situational awareness or contribute to the ability to concentrate on the most important tasks and objectives. It is easy for EMS practitioners to pull their phone out "just this once" or take their eyes off the road to glance at something on the MDT. However, these distractions, even when only a few seconds, can put the crew and the patient's safety in jeopardy, potentially leading to a fatal crash. In 2018, 3.2% of drivers in the United States reported using a handheld device while driving. In that same year, distracted driving led to 276,000 injuries from collisions. Does your organization have a policy against using a mobile device while driving? Employers could be held responsible for employees who are distracted or fatigued while driving in some regions.

In the Field

Another concept developed by the airline industry is the "sterile cockpit," which is meant to minimize distractions and help maintain focus on critical tasks. In the sterile cockpit, during key points in the flight, such as takeoff and landing, the sole focus of the pilots' attention should be on the task at hand. To apply this to EMS, when the emergency vehicle operator is driving, his or her focus should be purely on driving the vehicle. The emergency vehicle operator should not be distracted by navigating or radio chatter. This sterile cockpit concept is also employed by many paramedic services when conducting critical procedures such as rapid sequence intubation (RSI) where timing and drug dosing are critical to success. It can also be used for extrication calls or calls with the potential for violence.

- **Cognitive overload.** To overload is to give someone too much work, stress, or other difficulty. Overload can be in the moment, such as a critical patient requiring critical decisions, or over time, with stress building without the perception of support. It is often said that if something needs to be done, give the job to a busy person, but this is a dangerous tactic in EMS. The workload needs to be balanced between team members whenever possible. For example, an emergency vehicle operator should be focused on the road, not talking to dispatch or navigating. Overload might refer to task overload, emotional overload, or information overload. When a person starts to experience information overload, a self-protective mechanism kicks in, and the mind starts shutting down; if the mind is no longer paying attention, details may be overlooked. People can only manage five to seven things at any given time. Think of these as slots in the mind; once they are full and another is added, something is going to drop off. The more we have going on, the more we are likely to forget something or have it drop off our radar. Although we may not always be able to reduce the number of tasks we are juggling, it is worth recognizing that

the more things that are going on, the greater the chance of an error occurring. Sometimes a response to overload is a noncaring attitude similar to burnout. When this occurs, it is time to slow down the momentum ever so slightly and prioritize. "Okay, what needs to be done next?"

In the Field

Errors can occur when someone is task overloaded, so constraints must be put in place to prevent this from happening. A simple strategy is to divide the workload into manageable parts. This promotes teamwork, provides an increased margin of safety, and encourages strategies for handling overload. For example, think of the number of items you need to monitor with a critical patient: assessment, cardiac monitor, IV pump/drip, medication administration, patient's family, hospital report, and so on. Consider adding an additional practitioner to help you. Whenever possible, make sure you have the correct resources and necessary personnel.

- **Complacency.** Complacency refers to a sense of satisfaction that is accompanied by an ignorance of potential or present danger or deficits. In EMS, complacency can be understood as a false sense of security or comfort that masks possible risks. Basically, it is the idea that everything is running smoothly, so there is no need to check on things (e.g., all the equipment is usually in the ambulance, so I don't need to check each time). Of course, few people come to work wanting to be labeled as complacent. However, in accident reports, complacency is often listed as a cause. Complacency itself is not an accident cause; it is an effect. It is the effect of having a sense of comfort with certain routine procedures or practices. These procedures or practices are done so often and within the same environment that EMS practitioners often lose sight of their importance (e.g., "pencil whipping" the shift checklist). This is especially evident with safety practices that are allowed to go unchecked, such as seat belt use, appropriate glove use, and use of personal protective equipment.
- **Improper procedures.** Ideally, standard operating procedures (SOPs) are designed to keep EMS practitioners and their patients safe. Vigilance is needed to combat the urge to take shortcuts from those SOPs or do it "my way." Such an attitude not only puts EMS practitioners and the patients at risk for potential injuries but could also put the EMS agency and EMS practitioners at risk of litigation.

In the Field

A tragic example of complacency was NASA's space shuttle orbiter Columbia disaster on February 1, 2003, which killed all seven astronauts aboard the craft. The final report cited NASA's organizational culture as equally responsible for the disaster due to complacency and discouraging dissenting opinions. Although NASA is safety conscious, the constraints of having to meet the busy shuttle mission schedule led to more risk taking. A piece of foam had fallen off the shuttle's external fuel tank during launch. The foam struck the left wing, causing serious damage and ultimately led the craft to disintegrate when reentering the Earth's atmosphere. Pieces of foam had fallen off shuttles on other launches without danger to the crew. Although the occurrence had been raised previously as a safety concern, a sense of complacency was present because of the previous missions' successes.

In EMS, how might complacency apply to getting units back in service, getting back to training, or getting back to dinner or shift change in your organization?

If SOPs are not being followed, does behavior need to be changed or do the SOPs need updating? Policies and procedures spell out what EMS practitioners are expected to do in certain situations, and in some cases, they only provide a framework to achieve a goal or objective.

Remember, policies cannot address all of the subtle differences that occur in emergency situations. Experienced EMS practitioners must determine the best method for implementing procedures that are designed to help them achieve a good outcome and should not be afraid to consult with medical control as needed.

In the Field

In January 2006, David Rosenbaum suffered a critical head injury during a mugging in Washington, D.C. Firefighters and EMTs responded and found him unconscious on the sidewalk. He was quickly assessed and incorrectly assumed to be intoxicated and without associated injury. This complacent assessment and failure to follow protocol resulted in a significant delay in Mr. Rosenbaum's transport and treatment. Mr. Rosenbaum, a prominent *New York Times* reporter, later died of his injuries. The national media took interest in the case because it seemed to highlight the issue of complacency in EMS.

In the Field

One example of not following SOPs was that of a nurse working at Vanderbilt University Medical Center (VUMC) in Nashville, Tennessee, who made a series of inadvertent medication errors resulting in a patient's death and an alleged coverup. The January 2019 Centers for Medicare and Medicaid Services (CMS) Deficiency Report established that the hospital had failed to provide standard hospital-wide safe medication practices that could have detected the medication error and prevented the death. The nurse admitted to accidentally selecting vecuronium instead of Versed (midazolam) from an automatic dispensing cabinet in override mode. This is an example of safety controls that are in place to prevent medication errors, but which can be overridden and still cause harm to a patient. Medications are common in EMS, and safety checks should be implemented to prevent such a tragedy. Policies should include a complete medication safety check before administering medications. Medication dosage accuracy should be determined by doing the math and checking it. As the construction industry would say, "Measure twice and cut once!"

- **Unresolved discrepancies.** EMS practitioners need to pay close attention to managing conflict. In many cases, the conflict is communications based. Conflict can be a normal, helpful part of collective problem solving if it is managed correctly. This means ensuring people are heard, repeating the message back to ensure it was heard correctly, and maintaining respect among team members. If there are conflicting conditions, team members must call attention to the conflicts so that shared understanding of the priorities and goals can develop.
- **Not focused or "no one is flying the plane."** The chief purpose of employing CRM principles is to provide collective situational awareness to the team. Although CRM relies on teamwork, CRM is not team decision making. Every team needs an identified leader who can make decisions. Teams

In the Field

EMS agencies should develop concise procedures for unusual occurrences (TABLE 2-1). Having a detailed procedure written ahead of time and staff trained on these procedures reduces the likelihood of deviation and the resultant negative consequences.

TABLE 2-1 Special Situations Requiring SOPs

Helicopter responses	Weapons of mass destruction
Large-scale incidents	Large venues
Special populations	Natural disasters
Improvised explosive device responses	Hazardous materials
SWAT requests	Fires

TABLE 2-2 Error Reduction Strategies

1	Maintain a high level of proficiency.
2	Follow high-quality policies and procedures.
3	Speak up.
4	Minimize distractions.
5	Plan ahead.
6	Maintain situational awareness.
7	Use resources effectively.
8	Practice avoidance.
9	Limit redundancy.

In the Field

Maintaining situational awareness is a continuous process as the surrounding environment changes. We need to be cognizant of the clues that tell us change is about to happen—a large crowd forming around us as we treat the patient or the changes in the rhythm on the ECG monitor.

without leaders tend to wander among options, with no one person assuming responsibility for the team's actions or the outcome. "No one is flying the plane," occurs when everyone is too busy discussing decisions as opposed to making decisions. A worst-case scenario is when no one is maintaining situational awareness and/or managing resources. The team provides open, honest, respectful input, but the leader decides on the course of action.

Error Reduction Strategies

We have shown that errors are not random in EMS (or any other high-reliability organization) and that people cause accidents through errors. Errors can arise from poor communication, poor teamwork, not following procedures, or not paying attention. Pre-hospital morbidity and mortality could be reduced by preventing errors.

Personal Strategies: Error Reduction

There are personal strategies for error reduction, as listed in TABLE 2-2. First, maintain a high level of proficiency in your knowledge and skills. Follow high-quality policies and procedures by training on your protocols and SOPs to avoid discrepancies. If there is any confusion, ask your supervisor or medical director to clarify any protocols you think are vague or confusing. Have open communications and ensure that everyone on the team knows that he or she can call a safety time-out if things are not clear. Do not be afraid to speak up. If you see something wrong, announce it before an error occurs. For example, if a lifting and moving plan is not clear, you should stop before "Ready, one, two, three" is called to clarify your role.

Minimize distractions to allow yourself to focus on the task at hand and use the concepts within CRM to maintain situational awareness. Reduce the noise level, but talk as necessary. Plan ahead by knowing your area as well as your vehicle, and recognize any areas of weakness. Keep two hands on the wheel and your eyes on the road and maintain situational awareness when driving. Always pay attention and have an escape route. Use resources effectively. Wear your safety vest on the scene and block the roadway scene with your apparatus. Use job aids for high-risk/low-frequency tasks and conduct medication checks on all drugs. Recognize that technology has its limitations, and unless the equipment is properly maintained, it will not function correctly. Practice avoidance by avoiding (known dangerous areas, intersections, blind turns, etc.) as much as possible. Limit redundancy by creating layers of safety precautions as a fail-safe (e.g., drive defensively and always wear seat belts). Finally, accept that most errors are human errors, which is why it is critical to be a high-functioning member of a high-functioning team.

Job Aids

Job aids are critical tools for practitioners and can easily be created or downloaded to fit the service needs. Having a chart in the ambulance could serve as a reference, resulting in more accurate assessments and improvements in care. Consider downloading the following: a table of the Glasgow Coma Scale (GCS) values for adults and children, the rule of nines chart for adults and children, an RSI checklist following your protocols, and a table of drug dosages for specific weights and the amount of fluid that would be drawn up. Most regional or state EMS systems have downloadable protocols as a resource. Having such a resource to refer to helps simplify tasks like weight-based medication calculations when done under the stress of an EMS call or with decreased sleep. Interestingly, the rule of nines is the most-used algorithm employed by healthcare personnel. Despite this, studies report that in patients with burns that are 25% to 35% total body surface area (TBSA), the TBSA is overestimated by 20% by healthcare practitioners when compared to computer-based applications. This overestimate puts patients at risk for volume overload during fluid resuscitation. Multiple studies have also shown that, instead of 1% TBSA, the patient's palm excluding the digits is approximately 0.5% TBSA and 0.8% TBSA when the digits are included.

In the Field

The Glasgow Coma Scale has been reported to have discrepancies in application. A study reported that prehospital and hospital practitioners agree on the same GCS scores in only 32% of patients. The eye component was the most accurate at 74% agreement. The motor component was at 72% agreement, and the verbal component was the least accurate, at 55% agreement.

Data from Gill MR, Reiley DG, Green SM. Interrater reliability of Glasgow Coma Scale scores in the emergency department. *Ann Emerg Med.* 2004;43(2):215–223. doi:10.1016/s0196-0644(03)00814-x

Attitude

Having a good attitude is an overlooked error reduction strategy, even though hazardous attitudes cause catastrophes! EMS practitioners should control their attitudes and should beware the attitudes of others. Red flags for potential problems in this realm include comments like the following:

- "I know what I'm doing."
- "I'm better than anyone else here."
- "I've done it this way many times before, and nothing bad has ever happened."
- "I outrank you."
- "This is the way we have always done it."

Often these comments are made in high-stress environments and have poor outcomes. Anytime a safety concern is raised, it should be addressed. You may find that the action may still take place, or the order may still need to be followed, but when an unsafe action is recognized, it must be noted.

Effective Communications

Communication skills are vital to success in any situation. Communication is like a game of tennis (**FIGURE 2-5**). To be successful, both the sender and receiver have responsibilities.

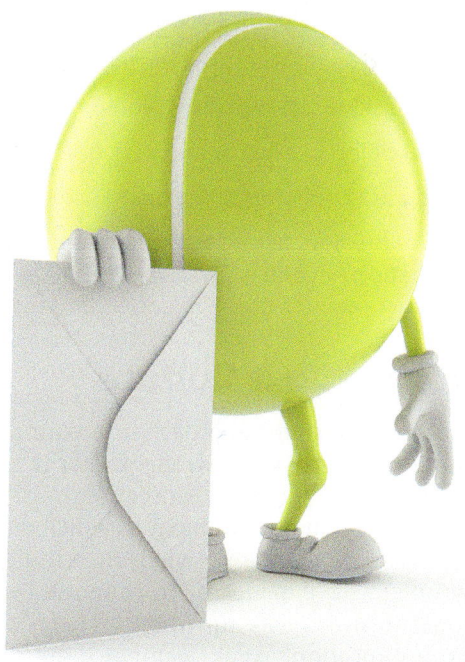

FIGURE 2-5 Communication can be like a game of tennis, with the tennis ball as the message going back and forth between sender and receiver.
© Talaj/Shutterstock.

Sending the Message

When sending the message, the communication must be clear, concise, and informative. There are many barriers to effective communication. Language, accent, gender, and rank can all play a role in how a message is sent and how it is received.

Receiving the Message

When receiving the message, you must: listen carefully and be receptive, confirm what is being said, and ask for clarification as needed. It is okay to ask, "Can I get clarification on . . ." Finally, observe the speaker's body language. Do not assume that all communication is spoken; nonverbal communication—posture, eye contact—plays an important role in conveying a message.

In the Field

When you are communicating, keep the following questions in mind:

- Did you hear what was said? Can you confirm what is being said?
- Did you listen carefully? Are you being receptive?
- Did you repeat back what was said?
- Are there language barriers?
- Is everyone using the same terminology?
- Are you asking the right questions?
- Are you being passive or aggressive?
- Did you ask clarifying questions?
- Can you provide an update if there is information anyone is not aware of?

Creating a Just Culture

Just culture is a systems approach to accountability. It brings a focus to *what* went wrong, rather than who is at fault. One of the intended consequences of just culture is to develop an environment in which employees feel comfortable speaking up when they notice something wrong or have made an error themselves.

We all need to speak up when it comes to safety. Poor communication, weak teamwork, and bravado are the top causes of line-of-duty deaths and injuries in the field. Most incidents resulting in injuries are predictable and could likely be recognized using a team approach. In later chapters of this book the just culture concept will be expanded and reinforced.

When groups of competent, trained individuals get together to solve problems, they typically define the issue and then deploy a combination of "humanware," software, and hardware to solve the problem. In this context, **software** implementation can be rewriting training manuals or procedures or developing checklists and policies. **Hardware** solutions can take the form of the use of computers, vehicles, tools, medications, or protective equipment. The **humanware** component consists of those people who are part of a team and have been directed to solve a particular problem—for example, a patient in respiratory arrest. EMS agencies with open communication and that embrace respectful and informed feedback as a method for encouraging collective situational awareness develop skills for their humanware to solve complex problems effectively within dynamic environments—for example, an ambulance crew working together to assess and care for a patient in cardiac arrest in the crowded chaos of a county fair. Essentially, EMS agencies that practice CRM build up the communication skills of their EMS practitioners and ingrain these skills into daily practice.

Simply embracing an open communication environment and encouraging collaboration does not address all of the differences in individual behavior and communication styles. An experienced and seasoned EMS practitioner who is part of a problem-solving team understands that he or she will make little progress if the human team members are unable to communicate effectively.

In the Field

The success of CRM depends on its acceptance by the entire EMS agency. To ensure that every EMS practitioner starts and stays on the same page, laying a solid foundation in the tools of CRM is necessary. This foundation includes training personnel in the techniques of open and respectful communication, developing a comprehensive approach to identifying and tracking errors and mistakes, educating and training personnel in conflict management, and instituting regular and recurring critiques so that members can learn from each other.

Situational Awareness

Situational awareness is an internal active evaluation process that goes on constantly, much like size-up. EMS practitioners must update their situational awareness constantly through the following means:

- Observation
- Communication

In the Field

When an EMS agency needs to determine who should be driving the ambulances, the decision should not be made in a vacuum. Safety managers may review existing policies (software), use driver simulation systems (hardware), and review driver performance under direct observation (humanware). They may also look at support agencies for recommendations on how to evaluate a safe driver—for example, an insurance carrier.

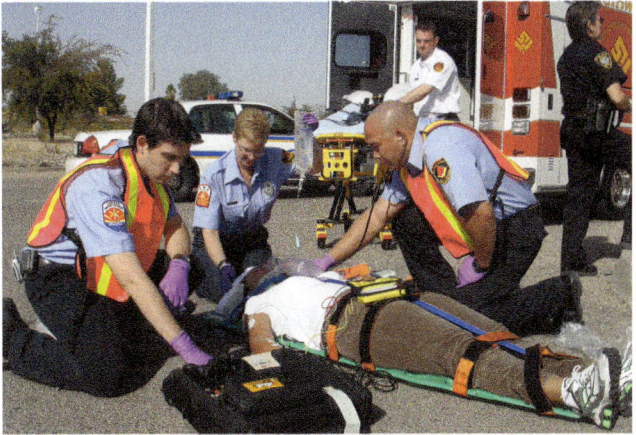

FIGURE 2-6 CRM is used by high-performance teams, such as EMS, to reduce injuries and accidents through teamwork and open communication.

© Jones & Bartlett Learning. Courtesy of MIEMSS.

- Alertness
- Full attention
- Perpetual vigilance
- Recognition of perception versus reality

Traffic accidents continue to be one of the most dangerous places for the EMS professional. Many agencies dedicate one responder to monitor traffic on scene and alert responders if traffic is getting dangerously close to the scene or if a distracted driver is approaching their workspace. Most crews have a "safe word," which when spoken over the radio is an indication for everyone to seek shelter.

There are three primary components of situational awareness:

- Awareness of the surroundings and how individuals are supposed to interact with the surroundings. A highway incident is a good example where crew are focused on patient care and not on the changing traffic patterns.
- The reality of the situation. You must ask yourself, "What exactly is going on?" Everyone has their safety vest on and the traffic is still flying by.
- Individual perceptions of the situation. Dangers are not just on the roadway! Beware the mundane calls, too. For example, consider a patient in a nursing home who is "altered." Don't assume it is due to dementia, as it could be many other things that might endanger you or the patient.

Teamwork

Within high-performance teams, regular use of CRM to gain a shared understanding continually improves performance (**FIGURE 2-6**). Specifically, when teams practice communication techniques that are designed to share understanding, members have opportunities to build team discipline, broaden the knowledge base of individual team members, and remove boundaries to learning. Additionally, CRM can establish trust and respect within teams, reduce the chance for error caused by distraction, and encourage collective situational awareness.

Because CRM is an interactive process, the roles of each team member must be clearly communicated. It is also vital to know who is leading the team. In CRM, although every team member's voice is important, and each person's role is vital to the team's success, there is one leader.

Team members should understand each other's roles and responsibilities. By "cross-pollinating," team members learn whom to turn to when specific problems arise, reducing the risk of one team member reaching the point of task overload. By sharing what their roles are with each other, team members become more likely to speak out if someone becomes overwhelmed by tasks or if they believe a fellow team member may have missed a cue that is important to his or her individual task and the team's collective success.

Conflict and Respect

Good teams develop a level of trust that goes beyond technical expertise. They actually come to understand the importance of collectively solving problems, and they value the diversity of opinions within the team. Diverse opinions, in any team, lead to some level of conflict. In this context, conflict is not bad. Instead, the success or failure of a team often depends on how the team manages conflict and whether team members are able to benefit from conflict by using it to outline strategic differences.

The trust developed within a team using CRM is based predominantly on the core value of respect. Every team member, when confronting an idea, action, order, or behavior, must exhibit respect for his or her fellow members regardless of rank, position within the team, or level of expertise.

Leadership Skills and Followership Responsibilities

Leaders can become leaders based on a legal statute or position of authority (e.g., EMS chief), or an EMS practitioner can assume a leadership role based on ability. The core behaviors of an effective leader are as follows:

- Envisioning goals and setting clear objectives
- Delegating authority and resources
- Taking responsibility
- Gaining commitment and motivating the team
- Maintaining situational awareness
- Understanding individual and team limitations
- Possessing the ability to adjust to the situation
- Valuing team diversity in experience and ideas
- Having the ability to listen and communicate clearly

In the Field

Knowing the limits or the strengths and weaknesses of the team and its members will allow leaders to capitalize on the team members' strengths and minimize the effects of any weaknesses. Lifting and moving is one example. If one team member has greater upper body strength than another, that will impact the positions that each member takes during a lift.

Most teams are created for a specific purpose—to get something done. The team leader typically needs to consider the number and types of objectives, their clarity, and their priority, with input from team members. Because there are often competing objectives and multiple methods for achieving them, effective leaders communicate what they perceive to be the priorities and then ask for input. They set a direction for the team. This ability requires the following skills:

1. Leaders have to model the actions they expect to see.

    A leader should implement effective resource management and use good communication as well as develop and follow organizational policies and procedures.

2. Leaders must be able to get the team's attention and hold it while distractions occur.

    Gaining and holding the team's attention can be done using hierarchy (the leader's authority position), but a leader usually has more success by employing subtle people skills. For example, some leaders have been very successful in getting and holding the team's attention by using steady eye contact and a quiet, calm tone of voice that requires the team members to listen actively. This method also can help reduce the tension level.

3. Leaders must be able to gain situational awareness, identify goals, and set specific and achievable objectives.

    Strong leaders understand that goals can be identified only after they have a sense of what is happening and what needs to be done. Situational awareness in a team environment requires activating a feedback loop: asking for input, requesting updates, and checking in with each individual. An important point to remember is that leaders should expect to receive unpleasant information if they openly ask for input. The news they receive may not be what they anticipate, yet it is critical that leaders maintain a sense of active curiosity, particularly if they perceive something differently from how a reporting team member perceives it.

4. Leaders must have the ability to ensure that all team members understand the team's stated goals and objectives.

    Misunderstandings are common in team communication. Good leaders desire a shared understanding among team members in which goals and objectives have a common definition. Leaders can achieve shared understanding by asking team members to restate the specific goal or objective. Questions such as "What do you think we need to do now?" help provide clarification, particularly if the goal includes multiple steps or requires the involvement of other teams for a successful outcome.

5. Leaders should share information. Often a decision is based on a lot of participation. However, that is not always known by those who are following, and this can lead to distrust.

Followership is a term for the personnel following a leader. Not everyone can be a leader; some people have to be followers, and this should not be taken as a negative sentiment. All good leaders have high-performance followers. The followers enable the leader to focus on the big picture. Followers also have

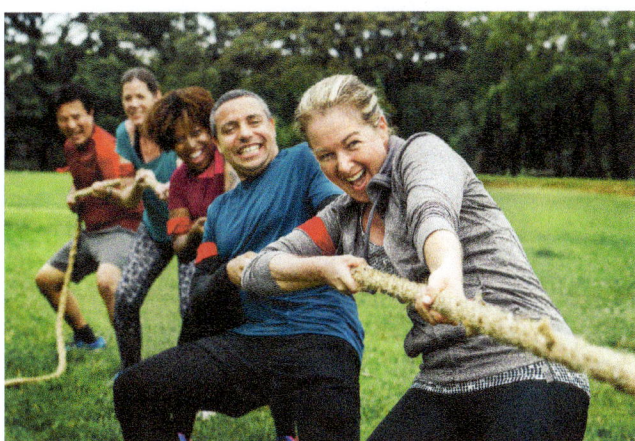

FIGURE 2-7 A focus on teamwork is essential for success.
© Rawpixel.com/Shutterstock.

a role to be prepared, engaged, and focused members of the crew. Just as leaders have responsibilities, so do followers, including these actions:

- Ensuring safety
- Accepting and following directions
- Being prepared physically and mentally
- Recognizing limitations of self and others
- Focusing on teamwork
- Having a positive attitude
- Being flexible

Success depends on the entire team, not just the leader (**FIGURE 2-7**). After all, it is the followers who will implement the leader's plans and act as additional eyes and ears.

Look at a typical emergency services organizational structure. There is a chief, and this individual sets the direction for the agency and sets the tone on the importance of safety in the field, with clear preventive policies and procedures. It is the responsibility of the "followers," or the deputy chiefs, to implement the chief's directions via policies and protocols. The field staff, who are also followers, actually ensure that preventive policies and procedures are implemented on a shift-by-shift basis. Without followers, preventive policies and procedures will not succeed.

Remember, a leader without people following is just a person out taking a walk.

Open Communications

The typical CRM model contains several key elements, all of which are integral to gaining a shared understanding in a culture of learning and mutual respect. These elements are inquiry, advocacy, conflict resolution, decision, observe and critique, and discuss options. In a typical incident, these elements are used in a seamless communication process. Once the steps have been practiced, team members often do not consciously walk through each one; instead, they use the process automatically, as part of the fabric of an open communication model that allows a shared understanding among team members.

The first step in the CRM circle of successful communication is inquiry. Good practices during the inquiry phase include aggressive listening skills, allowing an environment in which respectful commentary is accepted, and carefully intervening to ensure that the question is heard correctly.

An inquiry typically comes across in one of the following forms:

- A statement by a team member or the team leader: "This is our objective, to lift this patient up this staircase, and here is how we are going to do it."
- An order from medical control: "Give 50 mg of Benadryl IM."
- An action: A team member, leader or otherwise, performs an action that draws the attention of other team members.

All team members should remember that a statement is declarative. If a statement is made by a superior or someone with more experience or expertise than the team member on the receiving end of the spoken message, the receiver often misunderstands the statement as an order or a demand. However, it is important for team members to understand that statements are simply declarations of fact or observation and that they can still be questioned.

One of the most common errors made at the inquiry stage results from miscommunication associated with coherence. **Coherence** is associated with how well the receiver understands the message. Coherence is possible when the truth of a situation aligns with the words spoken by the sender. In some cases, the sender means one thing and the receiver hears another because the sender may be using terminology that is unfamiliar to the receiver or that has one meaning to the sender and another to the receiver.

In many typical CRM structures, the second step in the communication loop is labeled advocacy. However, advocacy does little to actually describe the process that occurs when a team member feels a disconnect with something he or she has heard or seen in the inquiry phase. Questioning authority is a daunting task. During this step, it is crucial for team members to understand that there are two methods for approving of an action or statement they see or hear, and only one method for providing a **challenge**. The two methods of providing approval for the actions or statements of others are to verbally state understanding and agreement and to voice no objection at all.

The second method of indicating approval, saying nothing, is all too common—and too commonly misused, as becomes apparent during **post-incident analysis (PIA)**. During critiques, team members might wonder how much understanding was truly shared at the incident. For example, a team member will state that he or she had a concern, or "knew" something was going to happen, but the person typically had a reason for not speaking up. Leaders are often astonished when they hear this. Why didn't the person voice an opinion? Leaders assume that everyone approves after they have asked for input and no one voices an objection.

Conflict Resolution

Few people truly enjoy conflict, yet it is a necessary part of team dynamics and a by-product of bringing together any group of high-performance individuals with experience and strong opinions. Add the components of personal danger, time pressure, and a high-stakes outcome, and it is a recipe for poor performance. However, it is not the absence of conflict that makes a good team but the manner in which team members handle it. The key to conflict resolution revolves around the saying "what is right, not who is right." **Conflict resolution** is a range of processes aimed at alleviating or eliminating sources of conflict; these generally include negotiation, mediation, and diplomacy. It is important to remember that CRM is not team decision making. Most teams using CRM principles are not formed on democratic principles; instead, they have a hierarchy related to training, position, and experience. It is critically important for team members to understand how they should handle conflict when it inevitably occurs.

A cardinal rule in conflict resolution—and one of the most difficult to employ—is for team members to stay focused on the mission or the issue at hand. Therefore, all participants must continually remind themselves to devote all attention to the current source of conflict. Conflict resolution is not the place to address past disputes. Biases need to be put aside. The primary goal is for everyone involved to concentrate all efforts on resolution.

When managing conflict at this stage in the CRM communication loop, it is helpful to understand that complete resolution of the conflict is not likely to occur until after the situation is entirely concluded, and that more time can be spent discussing options. It is important to remember that this loop often takes only seconds to complete in real-time situations. In the midst of any incident, the most anyone can hope for is to achieve an understanding of what the concerns are and why they exist. Sometimes the best that team leaders and decision makers can do, particularly if they are not planning on changing the strategy even after hearing the concern, is to communicate clearly to the individual expressing the concern that they understand what he or she is saying, recognize the potential impact, and value the input.

Decision, Observe and Critique

As indicated, the primary reason to employ CRM principles is to provide a collective situational awareness to the team. There must be an identified leader on every team who can make decisions. Teams without leaders tend to wander among options, with no one person assuming responsibility for the team's actions or the outcome.

One of the duties of a good leader is to take responsibility for team performance. Good leaders are decisive, yet they are also empathetic and careful listeners. A decision should be made when team members get behind the group's efforts, even if one of them does not necessarily agree with the chosen course.

During the next phase of observe and critique, team members need to provide input because the entire team witnesses events unfold after a decision is made. Additionally, leaders must keep in mind that during critical communication events, many decisions are made, and the constant flow of communication is critical. If a leader and the team have reevaluated their strategy and decided to employ a new one, it is imperative that the entire team be aware of this, along with anyone else who may be affected. Decision making carries with it a great responsibility.

After the decision has been made to move forward with a particular strategy, it is important for all team members to carefully observe the process and evaluate progress against the initially stated mission goals. If something appears unsafe, if things are not going according to plan, or if the individuals or equipment chosen for the task do not appear appropriate, a good team engages in critique conversation in which they evaluate the situation on the fly. This should be constructive conversation and should include specifics: What isn't working as expected? Why might the problem exist? What can be done to modify the plan? These brief yet important communications lead to discussing options.

Observation leads to critique, and critique should be an open process because it brings out comments, statements, and questions that lead the team to discuss options, guiding back to the inquiry phase. This is where good leaders shine: They encourage input, particularly when things start to get quiet. If team members are not commenting on their observations, they are not collectively sharing their understanding of what they see.

As the team members critique their work and its results, they may decide that other options are necessary. In critical situations that develop over a period of time, this duty is often relegated to a planning section. Within the small team environment and during rapidly developing situations, options are often presented as questions that are posed to the group. Options are a necessary part of emergency operations in any dynamic environment. EMS practitioners must recognize that even though a team has determined a course of action, team members must always evaluate other options. In this context, many team leaders start ordering resources and planning logistically to implement one of several alternatives.

Discussing options moves the team back into the beginning phase of the CRM loop: They had a plan, they made a decision on what to do, they evaluated their evolving circumstances, and they proposed options and outlined risk. The new option returns to the beginning of the process and is considered an inquiry ("What do you think of Plan B?"), and team members can openly agree with the idea or probe further to develop any concerns.

Decision Making

Emergency scenes are event-driven scenarios. This means that every situation unfolds in a manner that is relatively unpredictable and that the tempo of events is not entirely under the control of the EMS practitioners. In addition, each person viewing the exact same scene will have a slightly different perspective based in part on that person's area of expertise, level of experience, quality of training, ability to recall applicable procedures, and personal context. Members of any group on an emergency scene do, however, share two significant realities: No one knows exactly how the situation will unfold, and no one knows the outcome.

High-performance teams work best when they have a collective understanding of the situation they face. To ensure every EMS practitioner starts and stays on the same page, laying a solid foundation in the tools of CRM is necessary. This foundation includes: (1) training personnel in open communication techniques, (2) identifying and tracking errors, (3) training personnel in conflict management, and (4) fostering an open learning environment. Effective CRM ensures that every member of the team has an appreciation of the following key points:

- The exact nature of the problem, its cause, and any confounding or complicating factors

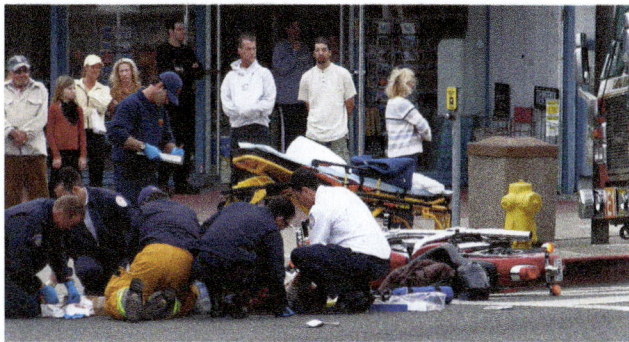

FIGURE 2-8 Unlike in situations where people have the benefit of time, emergency work is extremely dynamic and fast paced.
© mikeledray/Shutterstock.

- The skills, strengths, weaknesses, and experience of their fellow team members
- An understanding of what is likely to happen based on taking no action
- An understanding of what is likely to happen if the team chooses a specific action
- A shared knowledge of the desired outcome
- A shared strategy, with an understanding of what needs to be accomplished, by whom, and when
- The knowledge that any member of the team, regardless of training, position, or experience, can respectfully question the strategy and/or provide additional cues that will help the team gain a better understanding of the situation as it unfolds

Only when the team truly knows how to use CRM can it maximize the potential for a successful outcome. Gaining the ability to develop and cultivate a shared vision among team members is a skill that requires practice and knowledge of how the human mind works while under pressure to make a decision. Unlike in situations in which people have the benefit of time and know that an outcome will be the same every time they apply a set of rules and procedures, emergency work is extremely dynamic (**FIGURE 2-8**). EMS practitioners cannot know every factor influencing the emergency situation before they must make a decision, and they must be able to adjust and adapt as the situation unfolds. Team members should know when and how to slightly slow the decision process to gain a better perspective.

Errors Are Not Random

Errors are predictable, and situations that are predictable are preventable. In the 1930s, H. W. Heinrich, an industrial safety pioneer, reported on a study of accidents that he classified according to severity. Heinrich's report showed that for each serious-injury incident, we could expect to see that the same type of error caused about 29 minor injuries and 300 near-miss or property-damage-only incidents. This is commonly referred to as Heinrich's Law.

When applying the ratios suggested by Heinrich, it has been recommended that the focus of safety programs be on preventing less serious events as an indirect means to prevent a single serious event. Is it always true that serious injuries are caused by the same factors that cause less serious incidents? Many experts believe that this is the case. This is the reasoning behind near-miss reporting. If the factors that led to a near miss can be identified, then policies can be put in place to ensure that those factors do not occur again. Ignoring the lessons of a near miss will eventually lead to a serious-injury incident.

Risk Assessment

Through a risk assessment, EMS practitioners can identify specific work processes and perform a simple evaluation of the associated risk. To conduct a risk assessment, EMS practitioners first need to identify what hazards exist in the workplace. For example, driving with lights and siren, handling contaminated sharps, and loading and unloading patients are all hazardous tasks that EMS practitioners perform on a daily basis. Next, EMS practitioners look at each hazard and determine the potential risks associated with it. For example, with contaminated sharps, EMS practitioners would examine a pathway in which staff were harmed, such as being stuck with a dirty needle. EMS practitioners also need to look at the incidents in which staff are stuck with a clean needle. Next, examine how the needlesticks occurred: Was it during the IV attempt or transference of the needle to the sharps container? Was the ambulance crew provided with the proper education on how to use the device and how to safely dispose of it? Did staff violate the safeguards of the device or violate a policy? Was the device defective? As the cause is investigated, issues can be identified and corrected by revising training, updating policies, or changing the type of needle used.

A constant review by managers of incident reports, lawsuits, customer complaints, workers' compensation reports, biomedical information, fleet reports, and clinical counseling files may indicate patterns or trends that can be used to identify potential fail points. Once issues are identified, they can be corrected by changing a process, piece of equipment, or procedure. The corrective focus should be on those behaviors that can be labeled a high risk. Simply ask: How likely is it to happen, and how bad will it be if it does happen?

In the Field

NAEMT, in collaboration with the Center for Leadership, Innovation and Research in EMS, the National EMS Management Association, and the National Association of State EMS Officials, developed an anonymous system for EMS practitioners to report near-miss, line-of-duty death, and patient safety incidents by answering a series of questions in an online format. This reporting system is called the EMS Voluntary Event Notification Tool (EVENT) and is available on the NAEMT website.

The purpose of the system is to collect and aggregate data that are then analyzed and used in the development of EMS policies and procedures, and for use in training, educating, and preventing similar events from occurring in the future. No individual responses are shared or transmitted to other parties. The aggregated data collected are provided to state EMS offices and the appropriate federal agencies with jurisdiction over EMS on a quarterly and annual basis.

CRM Success Strategies

The success of CRM depends on its acceptance by the entire EMS agency. To ensure every EMS practitioner starts and stays on the same page, laying a solid foundation in the tools of CRM is necessary. This foundation includes training personnel in open communication techniques, identifying and tracking errors, training personnel in conflict management, and fostering an open learning environment.

Effective CRM ensures that every team member has an appreciation of the following key points:

- The exact nature of the problem, its cause, and any confounding or complicating factors
- The skills, strengths, weaknesses, and experience of their fellow team members
- An understanding of what is likely to happen based on taking no action
- An understanding of what is likely to happen if the team chooses a specific action
- A shared knowledge of the desired outcome
- A shared strategy, with an understanding of what needs to be accomplished, by whom, and when
- The knowledge that any member of the team, regardless of training, position, or experience can

respectfully question the strategy and/or provide additional clues that will help the team to gain a better understanding of the situation as it unfolds

TeamSTEPPS®

TeamSTEPPS is a teamwork-based system developed for healthcare professionals by the Agency for Healthcare Research and Quality (AHRQ) and the U.S. Department of Defense. It stands for Team Strategies and Tools to Enhance Performance and Patient Safety. It is an additional model that may be used by EMS agencies and personnel to improve a culture of safety. TeamSTEPPS uses an evidence-based system to increase communication and teamwork skills. It increases safer patient care with higher quality by clarifying team roles and responsibilities and increasing team awareness. It increases information sharing and conflict resolution. TeamSTEPPS, illustrated in **FIGURE 2-9**, includes five principles focused on creating and maintaining a culture of safety. The principles include the following:

1. **Team structure.** Requires coordinated actions of a multisystem team, which includes the patient, core team or contingency teams, coordinating team, ancillary and support services, and administration.

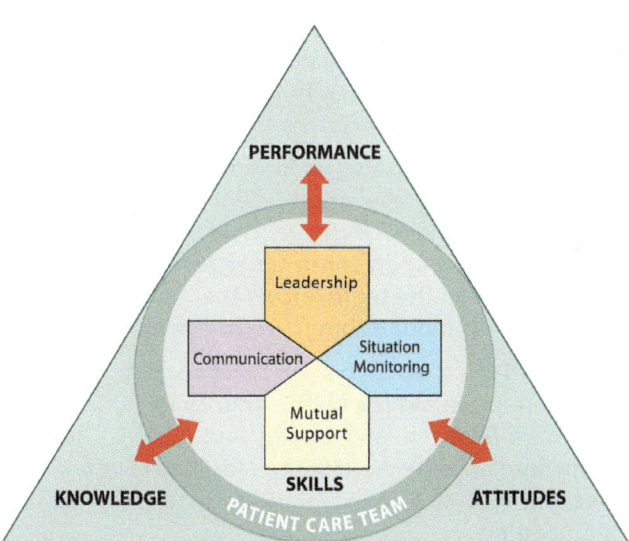

FIGURE 2-9 TeamSTEPPS is a teamwork-based system developed for healthcare professionals by the Agency for Healthcare Research and Quality and the U.S. Department of Defense.

Reproduced from Agency for Healthcare Research and Quality. Pocket guide: TeamSTEPPS. Updated December 2013. https://www.ahrq.gov/teamstepps/instructor/essentials/pocketguide.html

2. **Communication.** Stresses a communication process for all team members using SBAR, call-out, check-back, and hand off. SBAR is an acronym used to address critical information needing immediate attention and action regarding the patient. It stands for situation, background, assessment, and recommendations and request. The call-out is a technique used to communicate critical information to inform all team members of a critical situation. It identifies the team's next steps and directs responsibility to personnel to carry out a specific task. The check-back technique ensures that communication provided by the sender is clear and understood by the receiver. The steps include: sender gives the message, receiver accepts the message and responds with the message received for confirmation, and the sender ensures that the message was received as given. The hand off is the transfer of responsibility and information during care transition. I PASS the BATON is a mnemonic for a strategy developed to ensure a smooth transition of care. It stands for Introduction, Patient, Assessment, Situation, Safety concerns, Background, Actions, Timing, Ownership, and Next.

3. **Leadership.** Excellent leaders have multiple responsibilities to ensure that effective leadership is provided:
   - Organize a team.
   - Provide clear goals.
   - Assign responsibilities and tasks.
   - Monitor and change the plan as needed.
   - Review the team's performance and give feedback.
   - Allocate resources effectively.
   - Facilitate information sharing.
   - Encourage team involvement.
   - Facilitate conflict resolution within the team.
   - Model effective teamwork.

4. **Situation monitoring.** Continuous monitoring of an event is necessary to gain and maintain an understanding of what is happening around you. Situational awareness, as covered previously, is the state of knowing what is happening around you. The shared mental model ensures that team members are aligned with each other through maintaining situational awareness. STEP is a tool that could be used for situational monitoring. It stands for: Status of the patient, Team members, Environment, and Progress toward goal.

5. **Mutual support.** This describes an effective team that will assist all team members with completing their tasks. Everyone should protect each other from work overload.

CHAPTER WRAP-UP

- Crew resource management
  - Helps reduce the inherent risk of EMS
  - Cannot guarantee absolute safety
  - Is only one of many tools that organizations can use to manage errors

SUMMARY

- Crew resource management (CRM) is a tool originally instituted by the airline industry to optimize performance and outcomes by reducing the effect of human error through the use of all available resources. The goal of CRM training is to enable high-performance teams, such as airline or ambulance crews, to achieve and maintain collective situational awareness.

- When groups of competent, trained individuals get together to solve problems, they typically define the issue and then deploy a combination of "humanware," software, and hardware to solve the problem. The humanware component consists of those people who are part of a team and have been directed to solve a particular problem.

- EMS agencies with open communication and that embrace respectful and informed feedback as a method for encouraging collective situational awareness develop skills for their humanware to solve complex problems effectively within dynamic environments.

- Within high-performance teams, regular use of CRM continually improves performance. When teams practice communication techniques that are designed to share understanding, it provides opportunities to build team discipline, broaden the knowledge base of individual team members, and remove boundaries to learning. CRM can establish trust and respect within teams, reduce the chance for error caused by distraction, and encourage collective situational awareness.

- Situational awareness has three primary components: an awareness of the surroundings and how individuals are supposed to interact with the surroundings, the reality of the situation, and individual perceptions of the situation.

- Situational awareness is an internal active evaluation process that goes on constantly, much like size-up. EMS practitioners must update their situational awareness constantly by observing their surroundings, evaluating their options, and communicating with those around them.

- The typical CRM model contains several key elements, all of which are integral to gaining a shared understanding in a culture of learning and mutual respect. These elements are inquiry, advocacy, conflict resolution, decision, observe and critique, and discuss options.

- High-performance teams work best when they have a collective understanding of the situation that they face.

- Incident investigation finds that errors are not random in EMS. People cause accidents by making errors. Errors arise from poor communication, poor teamwork, and not paying attention. By mitigating errors, EMS practitioners can reduce deaths and injuries.

- There are personal strategies for error reduction. First, ensure a high level of proficiency in your knowledge and skills. Understand your policies and procedures. Have open communications and ensure that everyone on the team knows that he or she can call a safety time-out if things are not clear.

- TeamSTEPPS is a useful system developed for healthcare professionals by the Agency for Healthcare Research and Quality and the U.S. Department of Defense. It stands for Team Strategies and Tools to Enhance Performance and Patient Safety.

GLOSSARY

challenge More direct than an alert; when a team member physically moves into the action circle, prepared to take the next step of emergency intervention.

coherence When a message is understood by the receiver.

conflict resolution A range of processes aimed at alleviating or eliminating sources of conflict; generally includes negotiation, mediation, and diplomacy.

crew resource management (CRM) A tool originally instituted by the airline industry in 1980 to optimize performance and outcomes by reducing the effect of human error through the use of all available resources.

hardware Solutions that take the form of computers, vehicles, tools, medications, or protective equipment.

high-reliability organizations (HROs) Organizations that operate in high-risk environments yet strive to maintain a learning atmosphere so as to minimize chances for error.

humanware The people who are part of a team that has been directed to solve a particular problem.

post-incident analysis (PIA) An activity involving team members that takes place after an incident response. It reviews performance of individuals and teams while focusing on learning lessons that can be applied to future incidents.

situational awareness The state of being aware of what is happening around you and recognizing the potential for threats to yourself or others.

software Solutions that take the form of rewriting training materials or procedures or developing checklists or policies.

TeamSTEPPS® A teamwork-based system that stands for Team Strategies and Tools to Enhance Performance and Patient Safety.

unsafe actions Actions that can lead to errors, injuries, death, and destruction.

REFERENCES

Agency for Healthcare Research and Quality. TeamSTEPPS. Published 2019. https://www.ahrq.gov/teamstepps/index.html

Baker D, Day R, Salas E. Teamwork as an essential component of high-reliability organizations. *Health Serv Res*. 2006; 41(4):1576-1598.

Berger B. Columbia Report Faults NASA Culture, Government Oversight. Published January 29, 2013. https://www.space.com/19476-space-shuttle-columbia-disaster-oversight.html

Bishop T. *Preventing Human Error Study Guide*. Error Prevention Institute; 2000.

Gerstle CR. Parallels in safety between aviation and healthcare. *J Ped Surg*. 2018;53(5):875-878. doi:10.1016/j.jpedsurg.2018.02.002

Gill MR, Reiley DG, Green SM. Interrater reliability of Glasgow Coma Scale scores in the emergency department. *Ann Emerg Med*. 2004;43(2):215-223. doi:10.1016/s0196-0644(03)00814-x

Heinrich HW. *Industrial Accident Prevention: A Scientific Approach*. McGraw-Hill; 1931.

Helmreich RL, Merritt AC. *Culture at Work in Aviation and Medicine*. Ashgate Press; 1998.

Kelman B. The RaDonda Vaught case is confusing: this timeline will help. *The Tennessean*. Published March 2, 2020. https://www.tennessean.com/story/news/health/2020/03/03/vanderbilt-nurse-radonda-vaught-arrested-reckless-homicide-vecuronium-error/4826562002/

LeSage P, Dyar J, Evans B. *Crew Resource Management—Principles and Practice*. Jones & Bartlett Learning; 2011.

Lubnau II T, Okray R. Crew resource management for the fire service. *Fire Eng*. 2001;154(8).

Moore RA, Waheed A, Burns B. Rule of nines. Updated July 9, 2021. In: StatPearls [Internet]. StatPearls Publishing; 2021. https://www.ncbi.nlm.nih.gov/books/NBK513287/

National Safety Council. Distracted Driving for Employers. Accessed March 5, 2021. https://www.nsc.org/road/safety-topics/distracted-driving/distracted-driving-for-employers

National Safety Council. Injury Facts: Distracted driving. Published 2016. Accessed March 5, 2021. https://injuryfacts.nsc.org/motor-vehicle/motor-vehicle-safety-issues/distracted-driving/

Seshia SS, Young GB, Makhinson M, Smith PA, Stobart K, Croskerry P. Gating the holes in the Swiss cheese (part I): expanding Professor Reason's model for patient safety. *J Eval Clin Pract*. 2017;24(1):187-197. doi:10.1111/jep.12847

Emergency Vehicle Safety

LESSON OBJECTIVES

- Identify the importance of vehicle maintenance and inspection.
- Recognize the professional driver responsibilities of due regard.
- Differentiate common emergency vehicle collision causes and how to avoid them.
- Discuss emergent driving dangers and when lights and siren use is appropriate.
- Demonstrate risk mitigation processes of working in the patient compartment.

Scenario

It is a normal night shift in the city. You and your partner have just picked up a patient complaining of abdominal pain. The patient is stable and is going for his weekly trip to his preferred hospital. As the emergency vehicle operator, you put on your seat belt before starting the ambulance. Your partner sits on the bench seat and alternates between attending to the patient on the stretcher and entering data into the laptop ePCR.

It's a nice clear evening, and you are driving down a one-way street with the window down, watching the people on the sidewalk enjoying the summer night. Your phone is going off; your friends seem to be busy texting tonight.

Suddenly, a car crosses into your lane. You yell, "Hold on!" and conduct a rapid lane change while hitting the brakes. Fortunately, the lane next to you is clear, and you manage to slow and avoid hitting the other car.

Unfortunately, your partner barely hears your warning. Your partner is unrestrained, and the rapid lane change and sudden deceleration cause your partner to fly headfirst into the wall dividing the cab and the patient compartment. You hear your partner hit the wall with a sickening thud. You call out your partner's name and hear no response.

You park the ambulance safely at the side of the road, activate the lights, and call for additional ambulances, a supervisor, and the police. You enter the patient compartment and find the patient is restrained on the stretcher but has a bump on the forehead from being struck with the laptop and your partner is unresponsive on the floor. You immediately begin assessing your partner, hoping she is not too badly hurt.

1. How can ambulances be made safer for emergency medical services (EMS) practitioners who are in the patient compartment?
2. What can be done to prevent injuries to patients and EMS practitioners in the patient compartment?
3. How can emergency vehicle operators stay focused on the road and not be distracted while driving the ambulance?

Introduction

This chapter is not intended to replace driver training; the goal of this chapter is to highlight the areas of emergency vehicle operations that too often cause injury and death. The National Association of Emergency Medical Technicians (NAEMT) strongly recommends regular certified initial and refresher training for *all* emergency vehicle operators. This includes both a didactic course, with a focus on local policies, and a driver training course.

We live in a society that engages in many distractions while behind the wheel. In other words, too many drivers practice **aggressive driving**. These aggressive drivers are only worried about their own immediate needs, such as wanting to check a text message, and are not paying attention to what other drivers are doing or their own driving (**FIGURE 3-1**). This is why it is critical for emergency vehicle operators to be on the defensive at all times when on the road, especially when operating emergently.

Many of the hazards of the road can be reduced or eliminated by safe driving practices. Additionally,

emergency vehicle operators often have a partner in the cab who can help mitigate the risks of the road by operating as a team with the driver. This practice was emphasized in Chapter 2, *Crew Resource Management*.

This chapter reviews the best practices for operating a vehicle safely. Many of these concepts may be familiar, but it is always good to review safe driving practices and integrate them into your everyday routine.

Respect Your Vehicles Like Lives Depend on It

Without the ambulance, patients will not be transported to the hospital. In many cases, the ambulance is the home of the ambulance crew during every shift. For these reasons alone, it is important to have respect for the ambulance. It is a very expensive and complicated piece of machinery. Your vehicle helps you to make a living and aids in the treatment and transport of your patients. Failure of this equipment can lead to higher mortality rates in patient care. Respect your vehicle when you check it and always respond immediately to any safety and mechanical concerns such as grinding brakes, missing or damaged equipment, worn tires, noises or play in suspension, and warning lights or alarms that are not working.

Finally, respect your emergency vehicle when you drive it by avoiding sudden evasive maneuvers and by being aware of weather conditions. As a professional driver you should always lead by example by following all traffic laws when driving with or without lights and siren. The emergency vehicle should be a safe environment for all.

If emergency vehicle operators take care of their equipment, their equipment should function correctly and serve the entire ambulance crew and patients well. Ignoring minor issues, delaying repairs, and "pencil whipping" the inspection sheet will lead to problems with the ambulance. If the ambulance breaks down during a call, patient care will suffer, and the disabled ambulance may become involved in a motor vehicle crash (MVC).

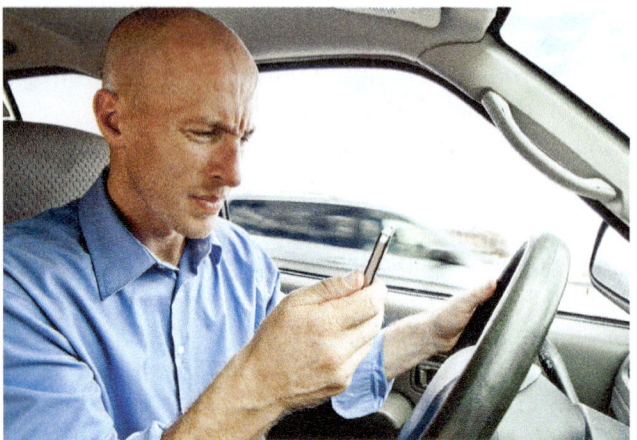

FIGURE 3-1 Aggressive drivers are only worried about their own immediate needs, such as wanting to check a text message, and are not paying attention to what other drivers are doing or to their own driving.
© becon/iStockphoto.

Vehicle Maintenance

Both the people and the equipment that help EMS practitioners do their jobs safely should be respected. EMS practitioners should get to know their fleet mechanics; it will help both the EMS practitioners and the fleet mechanics to develop respect for each other's challenges (**FIGURE 3-2**). The fleet mechanics can teach ambulance crews about the specifics of the vehicle and share the warning signs that indicate a potential issue. They also can help you know your vehicles so you can pay attention to what your vehicles are telling you and communicate when something does not feel or look correct with your ambulance. If there is a strong relationship between the ambulance crew and fleet mechanics, the fleet mechanics will be more apt to listen to the ambulance crew and investigate complaints about and issues with the ambulance. Get to know your fleet mechanics and always remember, mechanics are the people who "pack your parachute."

Vehicle Inspections

Ambulances are poorly designed for maneuverability, quick stops, and handling under excessive forces. Because of this, a well-maintained and routinely inspected vehicle is a crucial component of ambulance safety. Vehicle inspections should be taught, monitored, documented, and retained (**FIGURE 3-3**). Each EMS agency will have its own policies and procedures regarding what it expects ambulance crews to do in a daily vehicle check. Taking responsibility for your ambulance means performing an agency vehicle inspection. There should be a formalized list of items that, if present, indicate the ambulance should be taken out

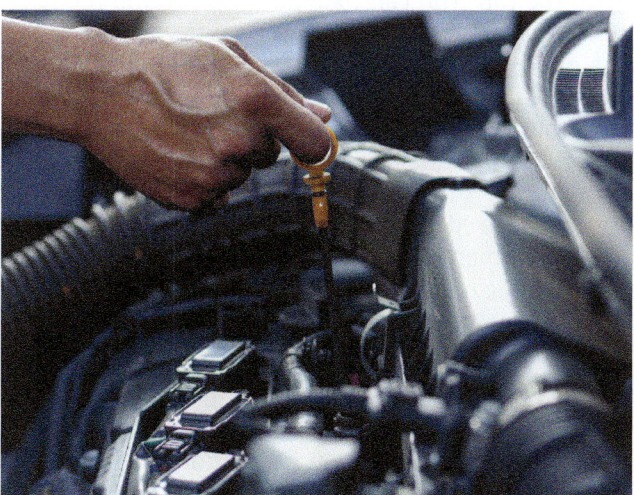

FIGURE 3-2 Show respect to all of the people and equipment that help you to do your job.
© ritfuse/Shutterstock.

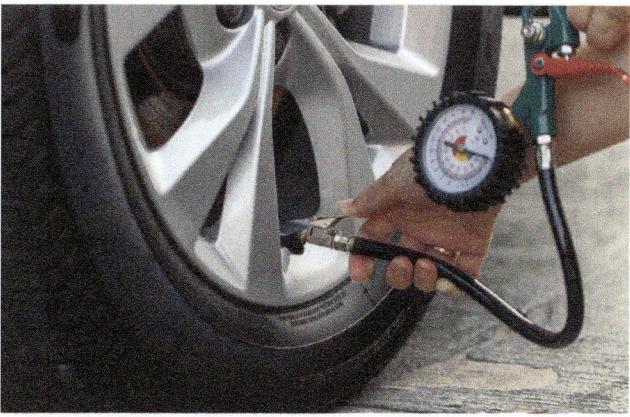

FIGURE 3-3 Vehicle inspections are a crucial component in preventing MVCs.
© wi6995/Shutterstock.

of service immediately. Crew inspection should include the following:

- Check oils and fluid levels.
- Inspect washer fluid and wipers (wipers in more arid regions may dry rot).
- Inspect for cracked hoses or small leaks that could fail.
- Inspect tires for air pressure and abnormal wear.
- Ensure warning lights and devices such as backup alarms are working correctly.

If crews believe that a vehicle is unsafe, they should be able to take the ambulance out of service until it is repaired. Crews also have the responsibility to report all minor issues before they become larger issues. An EMS vehicle should be a safe environment for the transport of the crew and the transport and treatment of patients.

Professional Drivers

Emergency vehicle operators are professional drivers. Anything that takes your attention away from the road is dangerous. Safe driving is not something to be practiced just some of the time. As a professional you need to commit to safe vehicle operation at all times. Your driving skills should be refreshed annually. EMS vehicle operators should consider attending annual continuing education courses related to driving safety, similar to keeping clinical skills up to date by attending clinical continuing education courses.

Reviewing near-miss ambulance incidents provides an opportunity for professionals to learn about shortcomings in operational habits before collisions occur. Professional vehicle operators also understand the value of reporting these incidents. While near-miss reporting is not mandatory in the United States or abroad, many agencies have begun tracking them as a tool to prevent accidents. A professional driver's EMS vehicle should be a safe environment for the transport of the crew and the transport and treatment of patients. The best way we can stay safe is to stay committed to driving safely.

Unlike other professional drivers, there are no hours-of-service rules for emergency vehicle operators in EMS. These are rules and regulations that govern how much rest between work shifts a driver must have. Most professional drivers are subject to laws that limit the length of a shift. Although federally mandated hours of service do not apply to EMS personnel, some states have enacted laws that impose criminal liabilities on those who are involved in a crash in which lack of sleep was a factor. These laws have been used to prosecute ambulance drivers. Tired, drowsy, and fatigued driving is extremely dangerous. Some agencies may have standard operating procedures (SOPs) in place to combat fatigue and drowsy driving. Studies, including a 2020 study, support that being awake for 18 hours results in the same driving behaviors as someone who is intoxicated. Being awake for 24 hours is equivalent to having a blood alcohol content of 0.10%, which is greater than the legal limit of many states in the United States. As EMS practitioners, we need to examine our regulations and work rules. Emergency vehicle operators are professional drivers and need to be recognized as such. Dangerous practices need to stop before exhaustion leads to death.

Due Regard

Due regard is the ethical, and sometimes legal, principle that guides first responders when operating their vehicles to ensure overall safety to the general public, including actions needed to prevent the possibility of collision or unsafe behavior. Due regard laws change with geographic location, although the meaning and consequences remain the same (**FIGURE 3-4**). The

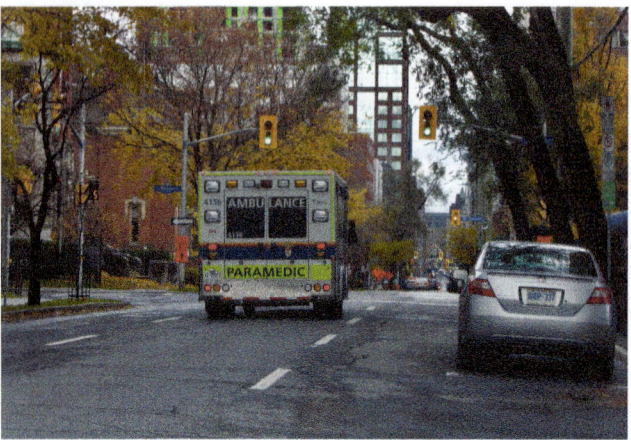

FIGURE 3-4 An operator driving in the emergency mode should give regard and attention to everyone else sharing the road.
© Masterpics/Shutterstock.

professional driver is well aware of the local due regard laws in their state or region.

When operating emergency vehicles, the responsibility falls to the emergency vehicle operator to not only ensure their own safety but also the safety of other occupants of the vehicle and other drivers on the road. Due to the distractions created by emergency vehicle operations, the responsibility falls to the responder to ensure roadway safety. Responders need to be familiar with the right-of-way laws for their area and the protections they do or do not have under the law, both criminally and civilly. It is important that responders know operationally pertinent local and state laws regarding safe clearance for emergency vehicles (also known as "move over" laws). Some states have changed from "move to the right" to "move to the closest curb." This is helpful on larger roads, especially one-way streets. Because the law varies from state to state, drivers may follow the law of the state in which they first learned to drive and not the law of the state in which they are currently driving. Never expect a driver to move a certain way. Be prepared to react to unpredictable drivers by leaving enough following distance and not closing in on other vehicles so rapidly that you surprise the drivers. Responders should know the laws and expectations of their area and bordering jurisdictions.

Defensive Driving

We live in a society that engages in many distractions while behind the wheel. Too many drivers practice aggressive driving. As emergency vehicle operators, we must always be on the defensive when we are on the road, which can be exhausting. Often, there is a partner in the cab who can help navigate around the hazards of the road. Remember, two sets of eyes are better than one.

As EMS professions, we operate in our own culture of aggressive driving. We can be aggressive, too. The problem is not just the civilian drivers operating around us. It is the EMS practitioner's duty to actively participate in defensive driving. The following are some recommendations for safe emergency vehicle operation that could save your life!

- Leave yourself an escape route.
- Use a minimum 4-second following distance for speeds of 40 mph or less and then add 1 second for every 10 mph over 40 mph.
- At red lights, leave room in front of you when you are stopped. You should be able to see the rear tires on the car in front of you.
- Be aware of your surroundings. Look out for hazards and road construction work.

- Look ahead and watch traffic patterns and traffic signals in the distance.
- Preplan and prepare some more! Ask yourself, "What if?"
- Give other drivers time to react by always using your turn signals. Make 12-second lane changes (4 seconds with blinker on, 4 seconds checking mirrors, 4 seconds to lane change one wheel at a time)
- Allow others to pass you rather than tailgate you.
- Avoid being closely followed to the hospital by anxious family or friends.
- Increase your distance from drivers that you feel are unsafe.
- Increase your distance in situations where there is poor visibility.
- Use extreme caution with multiple unit responses. If driving in tandem with another emergency vehicle, allow enough distance so that drivers will be aware of both emergency vehicles.

Most Common Causes of Emergency Vehicle Collisions

MVCs involving ambulances are all too common and costly (**FIGURE 3-5**). Approximately 10,000 MVCs occur each year, and this damages the reputations of EMS agencies and costs the agencies time, money, and personnel. These MVCs can cost the individuals involved their livelihoods, their health, and even their lives. The most common causes of these collisions are

intersections, vehicle speed, backing, and distracted driving. All EMS vehicle operators should obtain formal training in an Emergency Vehicle Operator Course (EVOC) or NAEMT's EMS Vehicle Operator Safety (EVOS) course to improve skills and learn about the four risk factors in detail.

The limited studies performed on MVCs involving ambulances show that a majority of the incidents occurred on days with no visibility issues and dry roads. This means that many human factors are involved, as compared with factors related to weather and visibility problems. It should not be surprising that a majority of these MVCs occur in intersections during daylight hours with traffic signals in place. This is due in part to reduced hazard light visibility, increased ambient noise of daytime activities (especially in large cities), and generally, more traffic on the roadway during the daytime hours. MVCs in intersections have the highest rate of severity because they are compounded by opposing traffic, side-impact collisions, and the likelihood of rollover due to higher center of gravity. Head-on MVCs are the deadliest types of collisions due to the increased inertia generated by opposing vehicle forces (i.e., a 60-mph head-on collision is equivalent to hitting a concrete bridge abutment at 120 mph). EMS vehicle crashes have a higher rate of serious injury than average vehicle crashes, and most injuries occur to unrestrained occupants in the rear compartment.

Mitigating Collisions at Intersections

Intersections are where the most significant MVCs involving ambulances occur (**FIGURE 3-6**). Fortunately, there are preventive measures that emergency vehicle

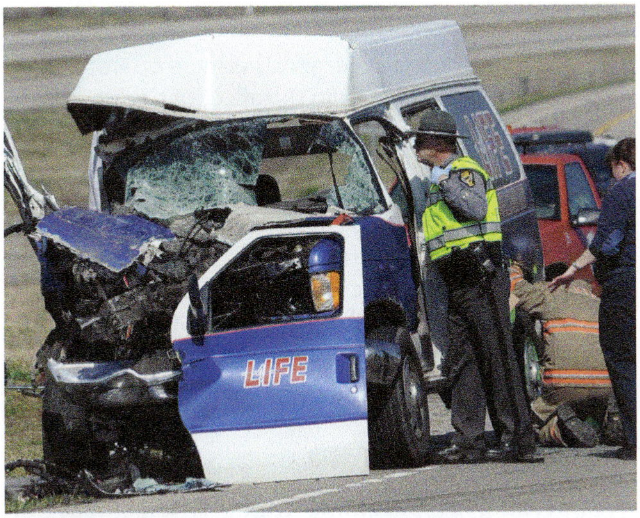

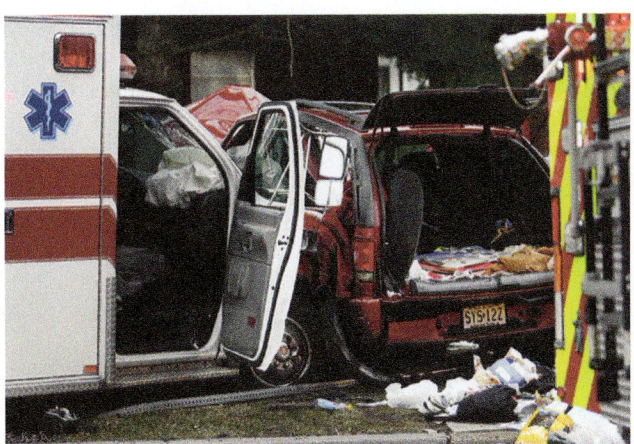

FIGURE 3-5 Motor vehicle crashes involving ambulances are all too common and costly.
© Frank Robertson/Chillicothe Gazette/AP Photo.

FIGURE 3-6 Intersections are where most motor vehicle crashes involving ambulances occur.
© Dale Gerhard/The Press of Atlantic City/AP Photo.

operators can take when approaching an intersection. As the emergency vehicle approaches the intersection, the emergency vehicle operator, or partner whenever possible, should change the siren's cadence. This will grab the attention of other drivers and alert them that the emergency vehicle is approaching. As the emergency vehicle enters the intersection, a secondary sound will also alert other drivers that an ambulance is near.

In any discussion on safety, it is important to mention that ambulances should come to a complete stop at all controlled intersections (red lights and stop signs) and then move cautiously through the intersection after verifying it is safe to proceed. Even though it may be legal not to come to a complete stop in your state, it is *highly* recommended that all ambulances come to a complete stop at controlled intersections while operating emergently. As the emergency vehicle enters the intersection, both the emergency vehicle operator and partner, when available, should be looking in both directions and clearing the intersection.

When moving through multilane intersections, it is important to slowly proceed through the intersection while clearing each lane. Failure to clear all lanes is a common cause of MVCs. Ensure traffic in all lanes has come to a stop before proceeding. Partners in the front passenger seat should function as codrivers. Stay alert and participate, especially in intersections.

Moving through controlled intersections against the signal presents a real danger to emergency vehicles and all others sharing the road. The same risk exists even in uncontrolled intersections and even when the ambulance has the right of way. It is important to watch your speed, slow down, change siren patterns, and even cover the brake with your foot in case a quick stop is required. Excessive speed through intersections increases the morbidity factor of many ambulance collisions.

If traveling through a green light, change the siren cadence, reduce your speed, and cover the brake pedal with your foot to help you quickly react. Never "push" other drivers into an intersection against a red light. If there is no clear path, turn the siren off and wait until the light changes.

Remember that yellow lights typically stay yellow for 1 second for every 10 mph of the posted speed limit (i.e., a 30-mph speed limit equals a 3-second yellow light). Crosswalk signals are a good way to judge traffic lights. Always beware the "stale" green light. Finally, Opticom usage may be helpful in changing lights or keeping them green as your ambulance approaches. These devices can be a hazard when running with other agencies or units using the same technology. This is one way that responders may collide with each other.

Speeding

The speed of the ambulance will play a significant part in the operator's ability to avoid an MVC as well as the severity of the MVC should one occur. As mentioned, excessive speed is a common factor in fatal collisions. In 2019, speeding was a contributing factor in 26% of all fatal crashes in the United States (9,047 of 36,096 U.S. fatalities). Speeding is a deliberate and calculated behavior. A speeding driver knows the risks and ignores the dangers. Excessive speed is not just based on the posted speed limit but on the conditions of the roads. As speed increases, the distance traveled before a driver can see, react, and complete a defensive maneuver or stop increases. When weather factors such as ice, snow, or water on the road increase stopping distances and decrease visibility, emergency vehicle operators need to decrease their speed to below the posted speed limits to account for the increased stopping distances. Speed reduces our ability to react. This violates the vow "first, do no harm."

In the Field

When traveling in traffic, the emergency vehicle operator should leave at least 4 seconds of following distance at speeds up to 40 mph and then add at least 1 second for every 10 mph over 40 mph. The emergency vehicle operator should also look 12 seconds ahead to avoid potential hazards and traffic patterns. These are minimum recommendations. When weather or visibility issues exist, these following distances should be increased. The key is for operators to give themselves enough time to react and to give other drivers a chance to recognize the ambulance's intentions.

Whenever the emergency vehicle operator believes he or she is in an unsafe situation, it is paramount to try to find a way out and take extra precautions. If another driver is racing or tailgating, it is appropriate to move over and let the driver pass and to create distance between the ambulance and the high-risk driver. One such situation may occur when a patient's family is following too close behind, or chasing the ambulance. A quick discussion with the family before transport should prevent this situation altogether.

Speeding in oncoming traffic is hazardous and reckless. It can be more dangerous in an ambulance because the ambulance weighs more than the average vehicle, takes longer to stop, and causes more damage if it strikes another vehicle. Some states do not permit EMS vehicles to exceed the posted speed limit, even when driving with lights and siren. In states that permit exceeding the speed limit, agencies should consider their own SOP to restrict exceeding the speed limit.

Speed reduces a driver's ability to react and increases the potential for traumatic consequences. An emergency vehicle operator who presses his or her foot down on the accelerator chooses to speed despite the knowledge of its potential consequences. Every EMS practitioner is taught that speed exponentially increases the kinetic energy that occurs during a collision and that by speeding, the chance of injury in the event of a collision increases. Speed reduces our ability to react. This violates the vow "first, do no harm."

Acceleration and speed can quickly remove an emergency vehicle operator from a potentially dangerous situation, but continuous speeding is dangerous, because speed is a contributing factor in an average of 30% of all fatal crashes per year, according to the National Highway Traffic Safety Administration (NHTSA). The reason used to justify speeding by many operators is the need to reach patients quickly. However, several studies have shown that speeding during emergent driving saves very little time and only makes a difference in very few patient care situations.

Many EMS agencies believe that it is important to have clearly labeled policies that limit how fast ambulances can travel. It is important to remember that if your agency's policies restrict the speed of the ambulance, the policy may carry the weight of law in your state and can add increased legal liability.

In the Field

Stopping a moving vehicle is a multistep process. The steps are the same no matter which mode the ambulance is operating in, but when the vehicle's speed increases, so does the distance traveled at each step. The first step of stopping is the time it takes to recognize that the ambulance needs to stop, which is called **human perception time**. **Human reaction time** is the second step, which is the time it takes the emergency vehicle operator to actually cover the brake pedal with his or her foot and press down.

The next two steps, **vehicle reaction time** and **vehicle braking time**, are not controlled by the emergency vehicle operator but rely on the vehicle to respond the way it is supposed to. In many cases, stopping depends on the vehicle being properly maintained. The brakes have to

activate, grab, and create friction to slow the vehicle. If the emergency vehicle operator is driving with the brake pedal covered (two-footed driving), or if the brakes have been heavily used, this may be difficult. The tires also have to actually grab the road. When water, ice, or other slick substances are on the road, traction between the road and the tires may be compromised. Tire pressure and tread wear will also impact the traction, which is why it is critical that the emergency vehicle operator ensure that the ambulance is ready for the road.

It is important to remember that these numbers apply to the average vehicle on the road, not something as heavy as a fully loaded ambulance. Based on the type and weight, the ambulance's stopping distance will actually be longer. Decrease your speed and increase the following distance in areas of poor visibility and adverse (weather, road and traffic) conditions.

Rate of Closure and Mitigating Speed-Related Collisions

Following distance and how fast an ambulance closes in on another vehicle can create dangerous situations. **Rate of closure** is the time it takes to close the distance between the ambulance and another vehicle, relative to the speeds of both vehicles. When you are driving in the emergent mode, it is important to allow other drivers sufficient time to react to the presence of the ambulance and to move out of your way. Lights and siren often startle people, and they may need time to overcome their momentary panic. Drivers can be unpredictable when an emergency vehicle comes up behind them and may try to stop or even turn into the path of the ambulance. If the ambulance is following too closely or closing in too fast, this may result in a collision (**FIGURE 3-7**). Assume nothing! Decrease your speed early enough to be able to safely stop if necessary. Emergency vehicle operators need to allow other drivers time to react and move out of the way.

Several regions have now changed the law from pull over to the right to pull over to the closest curb. Others have not. What are the laws in your state? Responders should know the laws and expectations of their area and bordering jurisdictions. Remember that people from other regions often drive according to the laws of their home location, so always expect the unexpected and leave a cushion space around the ambulance.

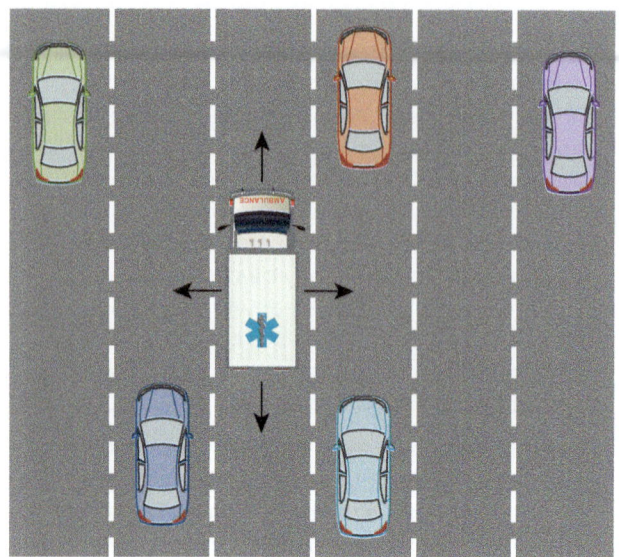

FIGURE 3-7 To mitigate speed-related collisions, you should slow down, reduce your following distance, leave an emergency distance cushion between you and other vehicles, and scan the road ahead.

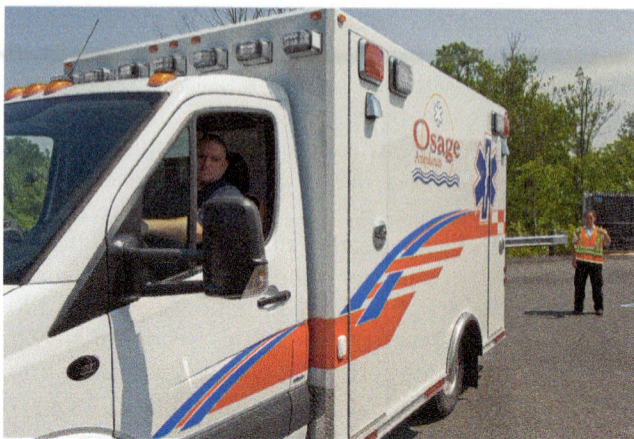

FIGURE 3-8 Use a spotter every time the ambulance backs to decrease the chance of a collision.
© Jones & Bartlett Learning. Photographed by Glen E. Ellman.

Do not tailgate! Tailgating is a common cause of collisions, even in nonemergency driving. According to the NHTSA over 2 million motor vehicle rear-end collisions occur annually in the United States. These crashes cause over 500,000 injuries and over 2,400 fatalities. Remember that your ambulance takes longer to stop than a passenger vehicle so you will require more distance. Leave an emergency cushion by increasing your following distance. Maintain a clear exit path if traffic should stop in front of you. Finally, scan the road ahead. Scanning will increase stopping distance. Because of the increased height of an emergency vehicle, it is often possible to see hazards before drivers ahead of the ambulance.

Vehicle Backing

Backing is an important space management issue. When possible, avoid parking the ambulance in a manner that will cause it to become necessary to back up. Operating in reverse, or backing, is one of the most dangerous maneuvers for an ambulance. Although operating in reverse most often occurs at lower speeds, backing is the cause of many incidents and collisions and even costs lives. According to the Department of Transportation (DOT), backing collisions account for 25% of all commercial vehicle collisions. The DOT also reported that 18,000 injuries per year are due to vehicle backing. Finally, according to the DOT, about 292 deaths occur each year from backing the vehicle. Considering that the average driver operates in reverse for less than 1 mile per year, these are alarming statistics.

In the Field

The children's advocacy group KidsAndCars.org estimates that 50 children are seen in emergency departments each week for accidents related to backing, and two children every week die from their injuries.

Data from KidsAndCars.org. Backovers. n.d. https://www.kidsandcars.org/how-kids-get-hurt/backovers

There are several preventive actions that an emergency vehicle operator can take when backing. First, do not disable the backing alarm on the ambulance. This is a warning device designed to alert people that the unit is backing and to stand clear. Even with cameras, there are blind spots when backing.

Use a spotter every time the ambulance operates in reverse to help decrease the chance of a collision (**FIGURE 3-8**). EMS agencies should have policies that require spotters while backing even if backing cameras are present. If the view of the spotter is lost, the operator should stop the vehicle *immediately*. If the operator shifts his or her gaze from one mirror to another, he or she should stop the vehicle *immediately*. While it may not always be possible to have a spotter outside the vehicle, if the EMS practitioner in the patient care compartment can watch at the back window, between the operator and the EMS practitioner, any blind spots may be covered without leaving the patient unattended.

Distractions

Driving is the primary responsibility of the emergency vehicle operator, and *everything else* can wait.

The operator must be focused on driving the ambulance so that he or she is prepared to react and maneuver instantly to avoid MVCs. The first rule of coming into work is to go home from work safely.

Distractions increase the risk of collisions. The full effects of distracted driving are difficult to document. The NHTSA confirmed that 3,142 fatalities were identified in 2019 as a result of being distracted as the primary cause of death. We have many "opportunities" to be distracted while operating an emergency vehicle. Driving is one of the most important and dangerous elements of the job. Our patients, partners, families, and the general public deserve alert and professional emergency vehicle operators behind the wheel of all emergency vehicles. Driving distractions include music, conversation, sightseeing, cell phones, mobile data terminals, global positioning system (GPS), and food. All of these distractions can be controlled. To prevent MVCs due to distractions, EMS needs to adopt the principles of crew resource management and create a sterile cab. Distractions need to be reduced to only the most necessary of equipment.

Visual distractions are anything that lures you to take your eyes off the road. This type of distraction can be caused by coworkers pointing out sights along the side of the road, or a GPS map that an emergency vehicle operator is trying to use for navigation. Even the mobile data computer (MDC) displaying new run information can create a visual distraction for the operator.

Manual distractions are those that cause you to take your hands off the wheel (**FIGURE 3-9**). There are several overlaps between visual and manual distractions. For example, when an emergency vehicle operator reaches for an item, he or she will first look to see where the item is and then take one hand off the wheel to reach for the item. Items such as siren switches and radios are manual distractions. Even marking status changes with an MDC causes the operator to remove a hand from the wheel and is a manual distraction.

Cognitive distractions take your mind off the road (**FIGURE 3-10**). Cognitive distractions can be both run related and non–run related. To avoid cognitive distractions, it is important to stop personal conversations when driving in the ambulance. Talking is not forbidden, but it should be related to the road, the scene, and safely arriving at the destination. Cognitive distractions are not just related to conversations; they can be personal issues that are distracting the operator. The emergency vehicle operator should be focused on driving, not what's for dinner, an argument with a significant other, or anything other than the task at hand.

Text Messaging

When it comes to driver distraction, texting is a "perfect storm." It requires you to (1) look at the screen and read a message (visual), (2) manually manipulate the keys to write a message (manual), and (3) think about what you are writing (cognitive). This means texting is a visual, manual, and cognitive distraction all in one. Texting while driving is also an example of a self-reinforcing behavior. Drivers get away with it repeatedly, which reinforces the behavior. But the reality is that emergency vehicle operators are unable to adhere to the responsibility of driving an ambulance with utmost caution while engaged in this highly dangerous practice. Data from the Virginia Tech Transportation Institute show that texting increases the risk of being in an MVC or near-MVC by 23.2 times. How many MVCs have you responded to that were caused by texting?

Many states have noticed that mobile communication devices such as cell phones have led to increased MVCs. Several states have taken the approach

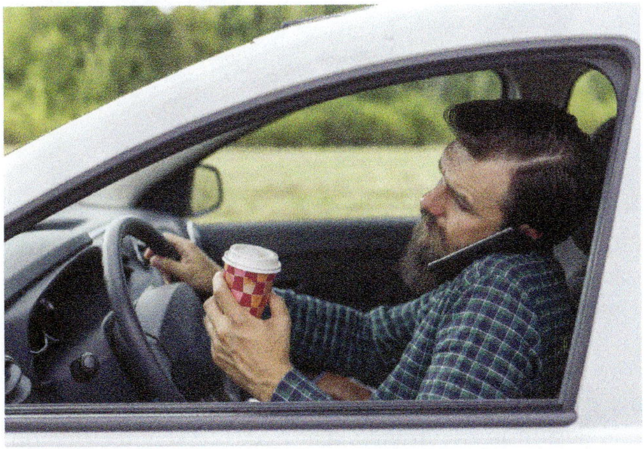

FIGURE 3-9 Visual and manual distractions can overlap and cause drivers to take their eyes off of the road and hands off of the wheel.
© Jinga/Shutterstock.

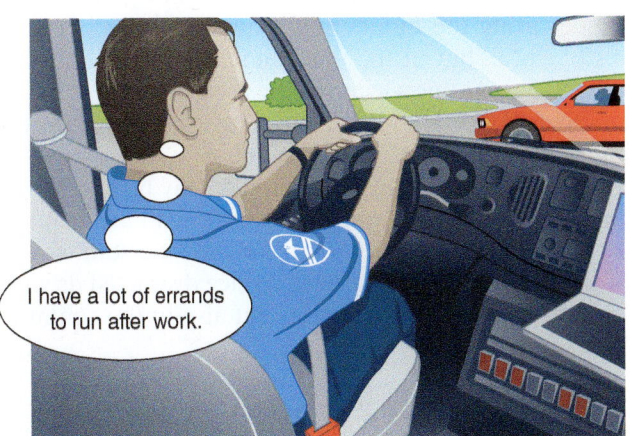

I have a lot of errands to run after work.

FIGURE 3-10 A cognitive distraction is anything that takes your mind off operating the vehicle.
© Jones & Bartlett Learning.

TABLE 3-1 Common Driving Distractions

Type of Distraction	Increased Risk (Times)
Drinking (nonalcoholic)	Even
Eating	1.6
Applying makeup	3.1
Drinking (alcoholic)	4.1
Reaching for moving object	8.8
Texting	23.2

TABLE 3-2 Ten Actions to Combat Distracted Driving

1. Leave your phone on silent and out of reach, and only check for messages when your vehicle has been placed in park.
2. Have your partner answer your phone or reply for you.
3. If you need to have a phone conversation or text, have your partner drive.
4. Secure all objects in the ambulance.
5. Have your partner navigate or plan your route before driving.
6. Have your partner handle the radios whenever possible.
7. Talk on the radio only when it is safe to do so—that is, before placing the vehicle in drive, at red lights, etc.
8. Place any object that you feel may distract you out of sight and out of reach.
9. Pull over to the side of the road if you feel the need to deviate from a safe practice.
10. Get a good night's rest and do not drive while drowsy.

of banning these devices at various levels. Some states limit texting and emailing while driving; other states have banned all devices without hands-free operation. A few states have attempted to ban all phone use while driving to eliminate distracted drivers.

Unfortunately, cellular devices are not the only type of distraction that increases MVCs. See **TABLE 3-1** for a list of various driver distractions and how much they increase the chance of an MVC.

The emergency vehicle operator also needs to know where he or she is going. Trying to navigate in unfamiliar areas can create a serious distraction and cause the emergency vehicle operator to have to look around for street signs rather than pay attention to the road. Using the principles of crew resource management, the partner should act as a codriver and navigator so that the emergency vehicle operator can focus on driving. Ideally, the emergency vehicle operator should decide on a route before driving. GPS systems that "speak" may also help the emergency vehicle operator focus on the road instead of navigating. Training in navigation techniques using the numbering systems or coordinates is also helpful, but in the end, there is no substitute for having a good knowledge of the area.

See **TABLE 3-2** for a list of ten things you can do today to combat distracted driving.

Do not forget that other drivers may be distracted. Stay alert and stay away from those who are blinded by distraction! There is room for EMS personnel and services to create programs to reduce distracted driving not only within EMS agencies but also in the communities in which they serve.

Driving with a Codriver

Following the principles of crew resource management will help the ambulance crew to share the responsibility of safe driving on the way to a call. Partners should be

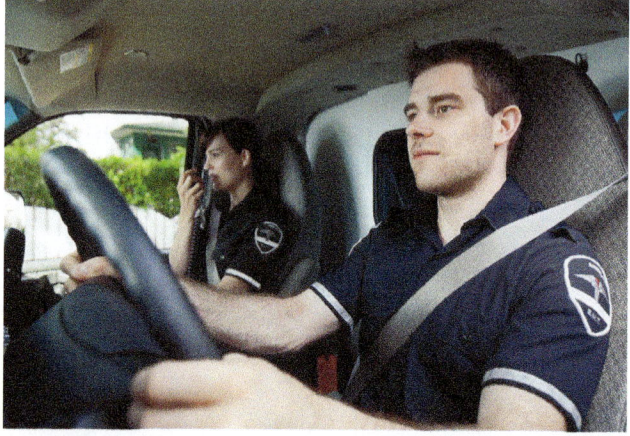

FIGURE 3-11 The person in the driver's seat needs to focus solely on operating the vehicle.
© Tyler Olson/Shutterstock.

communicating, double-checking intersections, and alerting each other to potential road hazards (**FIGURE 3-11**). The person in the driver's seat needs to stay focused on operating the vehicle. When there is a codriver in the passenger seat, that person should be responsible for nondriving tasks, including: siren changes, navigating, responding to the radio or MDC, and scanning for scene safety concerns when arriving on scene. Codrivers are a second set of eyes when clearing intersections while driving emergently. This can be a protective distraction, especially when responders in the passenger seat can reduce the risks of driving by staying attentive and engaged as a codriver. During patient transport, the emergency vehicle operator will have to perform all of these tasks. Limiting emergent transport is key to decreasing the times when a codriver is not there to help.

Codrivers can be considered a distraction—but a protective distraction, because a cooperative partner can reduce the risks of driving emergently by staying engaged as a codriver.

It is important that both parties know their roles, depending on which position they occupy. EMS agencies should implement policies that clearly define the roles of personnel on the way to a run. When clear policies are put in place, EMS practitioners will function in the same manner and have the same roles no matter who is paired together.

Emergency Driving

There are many terms for operating an ambulance in the emergency mode, including running hot, code 3 driving, or using lights and siren. Operating in the emergency mode is a significant factor in ambulance collisions (**FIGURE 3-12**). According to the NHTSA, 70% of ambulance collisions occur while operating with lights and siren. With so many collisions attributed to emergent operations, the obvious answer seems to be to reduce operating emergently. Studies show that using lights and siren does not save much time during transport, causes more stress, and is dangerous for ambulance crews. When operating emergently, everyone is at risk, and it is harder to perform patient care. A

strong emergency medical dispatch (EMD) program can help limit emergency responses by clinically determining who needs an emergent response for a potentially life-threatening illness or injury versus who can wait longer for an ambulance. According to a 2017 DOT NHTSA study, less than 5% of 911 calls are likely to have a patient benefit by responders running lights and siren to avoid collisions. That means that many EMS agencies could respond to less than 50% of 911 requests with lights and siren, and transport less than 5% with lights and siren. A strong protocol-based clinical judgment will help decrease emergency transports to hospitals by limiting emergency transports to unstable, life-threatening situations.

> ### In the Field
>
> Remember that the level of experience and skill among drivers differs greatly. Ambulances share the road with drivers who have variable skill, experience, and reaction times.

Think back to your last emergent transport to the hospital. Were you able to work and attend to the needs of the patient? Was the ride smoother than a nonemergent transport? Did the patient's anxiety increase? Finally, did the public quickly and properly move out of the way? In many cases, emergent driving is not very smooth because the public reacts unpredictably to lights and siren. This can cause issues with patient care and increases the chance of injury to the EMS practitioner working in the back. Also, the patient may experience increased anxiety from a rough ride, which could make conditions such as heart attacks worse.

Driving Risks to the Patient Compartment

Injuries can occur in the patient compartment without an actual collision. Have you ever been thrown around while providing care in a moving ambulance? Injuries can occur due to the following:

- Sudden evasive maneuvers may cause loss of balance.
- Curb strikes can cause neck and back injuries.
- Aggressive braking can shift equipment and personnel.
- Unanticipated cornering or sudden stops can be reduced by communication from driver to patient compartment personnel.
- Movement of the vehicle can result in slips and falls or spills of fluid from patient care.

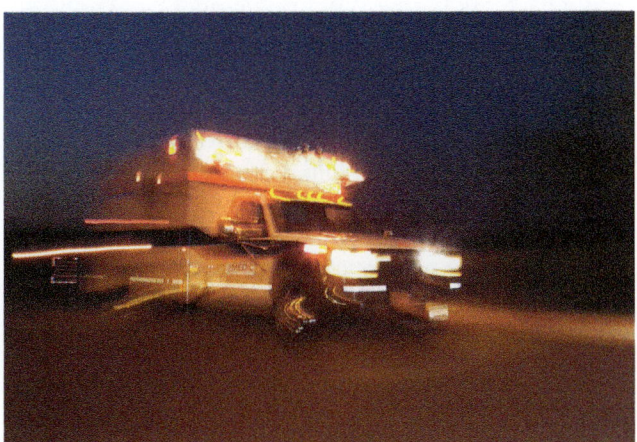

FIGURE 3-12 Operating in the emergency mode is a significant factor in ambulance collisions.
© Stockbyte/Thinkstock.

Dangers in the Patient Compartment

You are riding around in a box where it is hard to maintain balance, there may be shifting equipment or personnel, and the design structure does not always lend itself to safety. The risks of the patient compartment include the following:

- **Unsafe structural designs.** Historically, there were limited patient compartment structural regulations. Crash testing focused on the front cab area, not the back compartment.
- **Hostile interior surfaces.** Square corners on cabinets pose a danger to the body and head, causing injuries.
- **Side-facing seats.** Provide no support to the neck or back during collisions.
- **The need to be unrestrained to provide patient care.** Poor designs and ergonomics prevent patient care while seat belted. Responders become human projectiles in collisions if not seat belted.
- **Human and other projectiles.** Unsecured equipment and unrestrained passengers/personnel.

Ambulance Construction Regulations and Safety Standards

Making ambulances safer will take time, new standards, and considerable cost. Multiple agencies are working to improve the construction regulations and safety standards. The General Services Administration (GSA) of the federal government has released standards since 1974; the current version, KKK-A-1822(F), was released in July 2020. The National Fire Protection Association (NFPA) has NFPA 1917, which is currently under consolidation, with an expected update to be published in 2025. Finally, the Commission on Accreditation of Ambulance Services offers Ground Vehicle Standard (currently V2.0), which is accredited by the American National Standards Institute (ANSI) and created in conjunction with the Society of Automotive Engineers (SAE). As new designs and standards emerge, ambulances will become safer. In the meantime, actions can be taken now to improve ambulance safety—for example, using machines that automatically take the patient's vitals so that EMS practitioners can remain seated and secured with a seat belt while monitoring the patient. Before loading the patient into the ambulance, when it is medically possible, take a few minutes at the scene to perform such procedures as starting and securing IVs before leaving so that EMS practitioners can remain seated during transport.

Occupants and Equipment Restraint

The risk of occupational injury and death is disproportionately high for EMS personnel. Emergency responder fatality rates are 4.8 times higher than the national average. Many of these casualties are associated with transportation incidents. Simply put, ambulances are not built or used in the same manner as standard passenger vehicles, resulting in safety concerns for both EMS practitioners and patients. Although there are inherent risks to occupants in an ambulance, some of the risks can be reduced by properly restraining the occupants and equipment.

Seat belts should be used by everyone, every time, not just the patient and the emergency vehicle operator. The emergency vehicle operator should *never* be without a seat belt. In addition, any occupants in the ambulance should be properly restrained, including the patient and those attending to the patient. Seat belts save lives, and there is *no* excuse for not wearing them in the passenger compartment. Seat belt indicator lights and alarms should *not* be deactivated.

Stay in the Field

Seat belts need to be used every time. There is no excuse for emergency vehicle operators and EMS practitioners not to be restrained.

Stay in the Field

Surveys continue to show that a small percentage of EMS personnel *still* do not routinely use seat belts in the cab! Only 33% of patients were secured with lap and shoulder belts and as high as 84% of practitioners involved in crashes while in the back of the ambulance self-report not being seat belted. Practitioners and patients not seat belted are 40 times more likely to be seriously injured or killed during a serious collision. Emergency or not, *everyone* should always use seat belts while in motion. Remember, most EMS agency policies require restraint use. Emergency vehicle operators should take responsibility for ensuring occupant restraint use. Most states mandate driver responsibility, making the drivers legally responsible if their passengers are not secured.

Data from Cash RE, Crowe RP, Rivard MK, et al. Seat belt use in the ambulance patient compartment by emergency medical services professionals is low regardless of patient presence, seating position, or patient acuity. *J Saf Res.* 2019;71:173–180. doi:10.1016/j.jsr.2019.10.003

There are ways to decrease the chances of injury or death for EMS practitioners involved in MVCs. The first is simply to properly use the safety equipment provided in civilian and emergency vehicles. Seat belts save lives and increase the rates of survivability (**FIGURE 3-13**). Because seat belts have been proved to save lives, it is critical to consistently wear them whenever possible, even when you are in the ambulance.

Projectile Hazards and Securing Equipment

Projectile hazards include all unrestrained personnel and patients, patient belongings, medical equipment, personal gear, firefighting gear, and flight team equipment. All of these items may become dangerous projectiles during a collision and/or sudden deceleration or rollover. To the extent possible, store items such as personal gear, firefighting gear, flight team equipment, and patient belongings in an exterior compartment. All items stored in the patient compartment (i.e., patient belongings and medical equipment) must be secured (**FIGURE 3-14**).

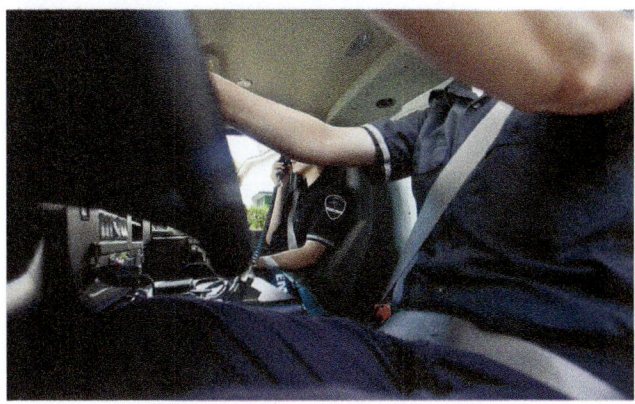

FIGURE 3-13 Seat belts save lives.
© Montgomery Martin/Alamy.

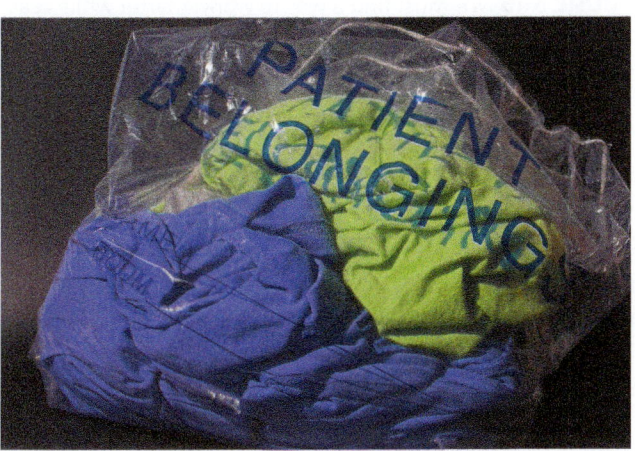
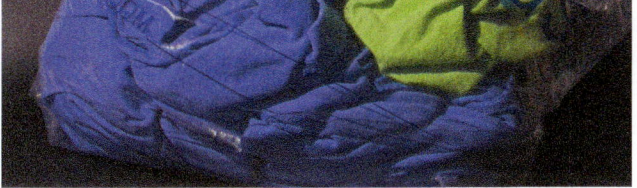

A

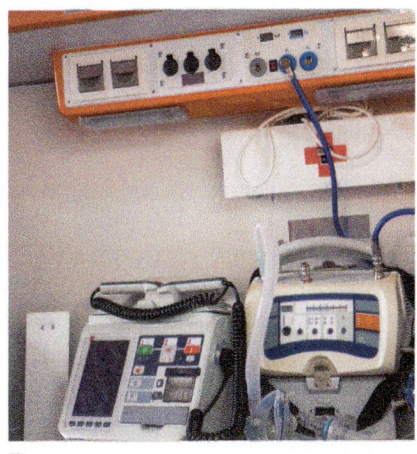

B

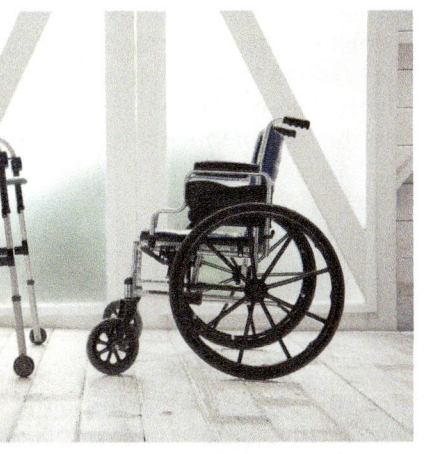

C

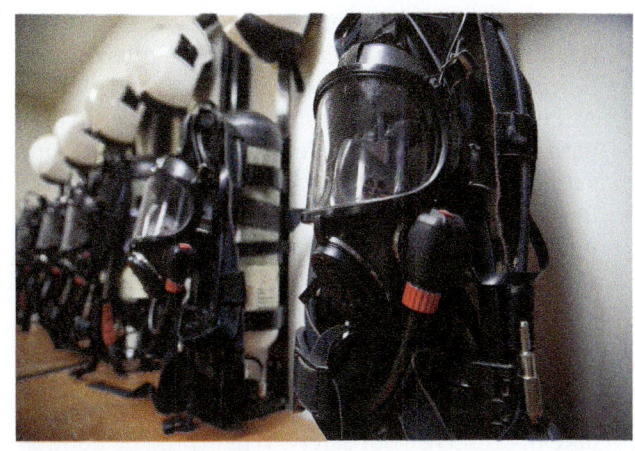

D

FIGURE 3-14 All items that could become projectiles need to be secured.
A. © Rob Byron/Shutterstock; **B.** © Zyabich/Shutterstock; **C.** © Erickson Stock/Shutterstock; **D.** © curraheeshutter/Shutterstock.

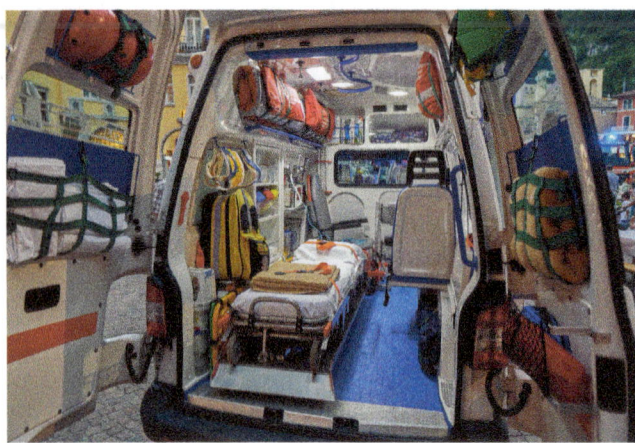

FIGURE 3-15 All equipment should have its place and be properly secured.

© Danny Iacob/Shutterstock.

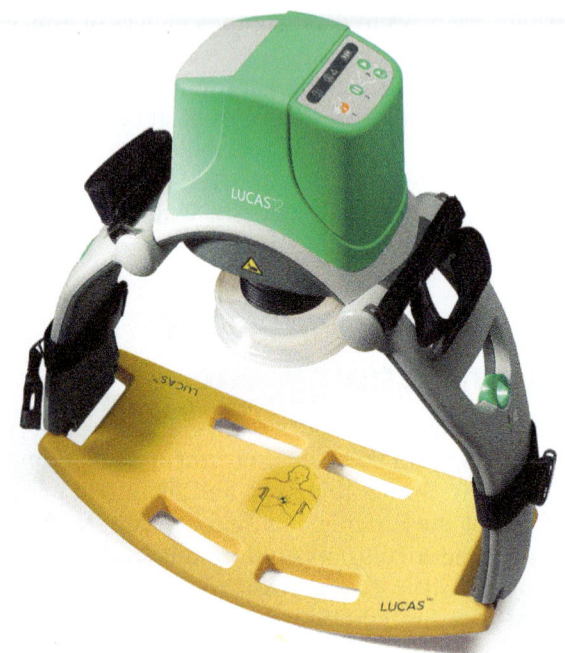

FIGURE 3-16 We must find a way to work smarter while seat belted when the ambulance is in motion. Shown here is a Lucas 2 device designed to deliver CPR compressions during transport.

Courtesy of Physio-Control, Inc.

Ensure that all normal daily equipment has its place and is secured (**FIGURE 3-15**). Review this list of securing equipment *do* items:

- Ensure that all normal daily equipment has its place and is routinely secured.
- Use cabinets, straps, and brackets to secure items.
- Secure needed equipment within reach whenever possible.
- Select soft kits over hard for the patient care compartment.
- Stow unnecessary items in exterior compartments.
- Use seat belts or straps to secure "surprise" items (i.e., patient walkers, wheelchairs, child car seats, etc.).
- Preplanning avoids last minute confusion or complacency.

Review this list of securing equipment *don't* items:

- Leave hard or heavy items unsecured while in motion.
- Have unnecessary items in the patient care compartment.
- Attempt to secure monitors and oxygen bottles with the restraints that are intended to secure your patient.
- Become complacent or ignore the fact that laptops, portable radios, and other small, hard items can become deadly projectiles.

Working in Motion

Consider the preparation and ergonomic actions you can take to preserve your safety. What could be done to minimize the risks while the ambulance is in motion? First of all, avoid driving emergently with unrestrained personnel. The minutes saved are not worth the increased risk for the patient or practitioners. Are there patient care procedures that could be completed prior to setting the ambulance in motion (e.g., establish IV, administer medication)? What equipment and supplies could be placed within reach to limit the need to move from your seat (i.e., monitor, medications, airway adjuncts)? What unnecessary actions could be eliminated while in motion in order to stay seated? Complete the assessment prior to going in motion. Perform compressions using a mechanical device (**FIGURE 3-16**). EMS practitioners must find a way to work smarter while seat belted when the ambulance is in motion. Unfortunately, caring for a patient in the back of a moving ambulance does not grant the EMS practitioner immunity from the laws of kinematics during an MVC.

Helmets

A growing trend is to outfit ambulance crews with helmets (**FIGURE 3-17**). These helmets could increase safety on scene and during transport. European and Australian ambulance services require that lightweight helmets be worn in the patient care compartment. With some studies showing that around 65% of fatal accidents involve head injury, it is important to examine the potential injury reduction a helmet could provide.

To be helpful, the helmet would have to be lightweight and not have any tails or protrusions that could

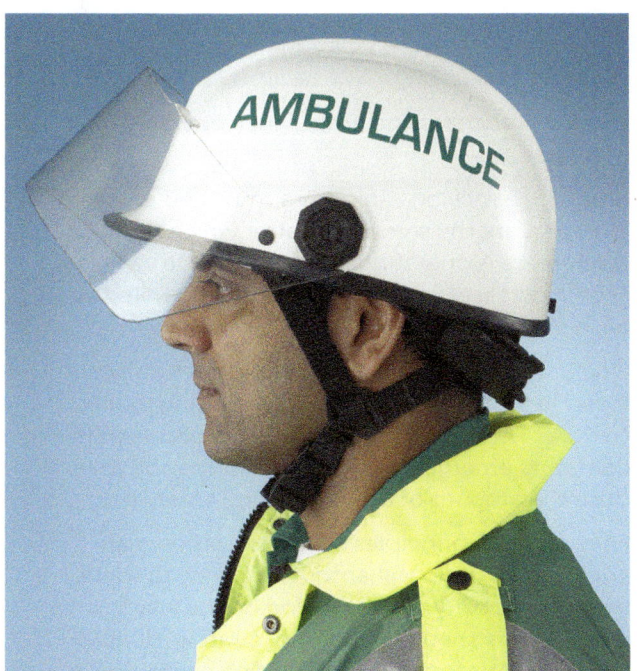

FIGURE 3-17 Helmets could increase safety for EMS practitioners on scene and during transport.
© Volt Collection/Shutterstock.

cause a neck injury in a collision. The National Fire Protection Association's standard NFPA 1901: Standard for Automotive Fire Apparatus, states that structural firefighting helmets are not to be used in vehicles because of their shape and weight. It is also important that the helmet not limit the vision of the emergency vehicle operator.

It is worth examining the benefits of helmet use given that our goal is to do whatever is possible to decrease injuries and deaths of EMS practitioners. It will take a change in the culture of EMS, but if EMS practitioners see that helmets can save lives, they should be willing to accept the change.

Patient Compartment Risk Mitigation

Failure to use the provided restraint systems creates risks for all occupants, whether personally restrained or not. Some important strategies for minimizing the risks related to collisions and noncollisions include the following:

- Use restraints whenever possible for responders and patients.
- Use a rear-facing jump seat when possible.
- Avoid standing.
- Allow only necessary occupants in the patient compartment. Unnecessary family or friends could drive in another vehicle.
- Consider "hands-off" patient care and communications technology that can provide more consistent care for the patient and would be safer for the practitioner and patient in a collision.

CHAPTER WRAP-UP

- Respect your vehicle and safety equipment.
- When operating emergency vehicles, drive with due regard using defensive driving techniques.
- Avoid common emergency vehicle accidents.
- Use caution while driving emergently.
- Be mindful of patient compartment risks.

SUMMARY

- The ambulance is the only piece of equipment that is used on every call, yet EMS spends the least amount of time acquiring, assessing, and maintaining proficiency.

- Because too many drivers practice aggressive driving, emergency vehicle operators need to drive with due regard and drive with concern for others on and around the roadway.

- Many of the hazards of the road can be reduced or eliminated by safe driving practices.

- Approximately 10,000 MVCs occur each year, which costs EMS agencies time, money, and personnel. These MVCs can cost the individuals involved their livelihoods, their health, and even their lives.

- The data on MVCs involving emergency vehicles show that four situations create the highest risks for

(continued)

SUMMARY (continued)

collision: (1) intersections, (2) following distances, (3) vehicle speed, and (4) distractions.

- The emergency vehicle operator can take preventive measures at intersections, including changing the siren's cadence, stopping at all controlled intersections, and stopping and clearing each lane of travel in multilane intersections. Becoming complacent at any intersection can lead to an MVC.

- Following distance and how fast an ambulance closes in on another vehicle can create dangerous situations. When driving in the emergent mode, it is important to allow other drivers to react to the presence of the ambulance.

- The speed of the ambulance will play a significant role in the emergency vehicle operator's ability to avoid an MVC as well as the severity of the MVC should one occur. As speed increases, the distance traveled before a driver can see, react, and complete a defensive maneuver or stop increases.

- Distractions increase the risk of collisions. Distractions need to be reduced to only the most necessary equipment.

- Texting is a perfect storm of distractions. It requires you to look at the screen and read a message, manually manipulate the keys to write a message, and think about what you are writing. This means that texting is a visual, manual, and cognitive distraction all in one.

- Data from the Virginia Tech Transportation Institute show that texting increases the risk of being in an MVC or near-MVC 23.2 times.

- Operating in reverse or backing is one of the most dangerous maneuvers for an ambulance. There are several preventive actions that an emergency vehicle operator can take, including activating the backing alarm on the ambulance and using a spotter every time the ambulance operates in reverse.

- Stopping a moving vehicle is a multistep process. The steps are the same no matter which mode the ambulance is operating in, but when the vehicle's speed increases, so does the distance traveled at each step.

- Operating in the emergency mode is a significant factor in ambulance collisions. According to the NHTSA, 70% of ambulance collisions occur while operating emergently. One solution may be to reduce the amount of time operating emergently.

- Following the principles of crew resource management will help the ambulance crew to share the responsibility of safe driving on the way to a call. Partners should be communicating, double-checking intersections, and alerting each other to potential road hazards.

- Emergency vehicle operators should plan their routes before driving. Partners should be used to help navigate to the scene whenever possible.

- A well-maintained and routinely inspected vehicle is a crucial component of ambulance safety. Vehicle inspections should be taught, monitored, documented, and retained.

- Seat belts should be used by everyone, every time. The emergency vehicle operator should *never* be without a seat belt. In addition, any occupants in the ambulance should be properly restrained, including the patient and, if possible, those attending to the patient.

- All equipment needs to be completely secured or tied down. Monitors, patient report computers, and other unsecured equipment can become missiles during MVCs or sudden evasive maneuvers. All cabinets should be locked and stay closed.

GLOSSARY

aggressive driving Operating a vehicle with aggressive actions, without concern for other drivers.

cognitive distractions Distractions that take the emergency vehicle operator's mind off the road and operation of the vehicle.

due regard The ethical, and sometimes legal, principle that guides vehicle operators to ensure overall safety to the general public, including actions needed to prevent the possibility of collision or unsafe behavior.

human perception time The rate at which a person perceives incoming stimuli.

human reaction time The time it takes for a person to react to an impending event.

manual distractions Distractions that cause the emergency vehicle operator to take a hand off the ambulance steering wheel.

rate of closure The speed at which one vehicle overtakes another.

vehicle braking time The time it takes for the vehicle to stop.

vehicle reaction time The time between when the brake pedal is applied and when the brakes start working.

visual distractions Distractions that take the emergency vehicle operator's eyes off the road.

REFERENCES

Ambulance History Injury Statistics and Standards. YouTube. Accessed April 6, 2021. https://www.youtube.com/watch?v=fKa0yWfhvGs

Ambulances Crash at New York City Intersection. YouTube. Accessed April 6, 2021. https://www.youtube.com/watch?v=T9bQRD AIrMg

Auerbach P, Morris J Jr, Phillips J Jr, Redlinger S, Vaughn W. An analysis of ambulance accidents in Tennessee. *JAMA*. 1987;258(11):1487-1490.

Beckera LR, Zaloshnjaa E, Levickb N, Lic G, Millera T. Relative risk of injury and death in ambulances and other emergency vehicles. *ScienceDirect*. 2003;35(6):941-948.

Braun Ambulance Crash Testing - June 2016 Compilation. YouTube. Accessed April 7, 2021. https://www.youtube.com/watch?v =QjLs2sUcw-M&list=RDCMUCZFEAilNmuR3KrHoUiTvWMg &index=4

Brown L, Hunt R, Whitney C, Addario M, Hogue T. Do warning lights and sirens reduce ambulance response times? *Prehosp Emerg Care*. 2000;4(1):70-74.

Centers for Disease Control and Prevention. Drowsy Driving: Sleep and Sleep Disorders. Reviewed March 21, 2017. Accessed November 16, 2021. https://www.cdc.gov/sleep/about_sleep /drowsy_driving.html

Currin A. Distracted driving. NHTSA. Published November 5, 2018. Accessed April 6, 2021. https://www.nhtsa.gov /risky-driving/distracted-driving

Custalow CB, Gravitz CS. Emergency medical vehicle collisions and potential for preventive intervention. *Prehosp Emerg Care*. 2004;8(2):175-184.

East Cambridgeshire District Council. *Accident/Near Miss Reporting Policy*. East Cambridgeshire District Council; 2017. https:// www.eastcambs.gov.uk/sites/default/files/agendas/rs270616 _R36Ap1.pdf

Elling B, Raheb R. *EMS Vehicle Operator Safety*. Jones & Bartlett Learning; 2017.

Elling R. Dispelling myths on ambulance accidents. *JEMS*. 1989; 14(7):60-64.

Federal Motor Carrier Safety Administration. CMV Driving Tips: Following Too Closely. FMCSA. Accessed April 7, 2021. https://www.fmcsa.dot.gov/safety/driver-safety/cmv -driving-tips-following-too-closely

Hunt R, Brown L, Cabinum E, et al. Is ambulance transport time with lights and sirens faster than that without? *Ann Emerg Med*. 1995;25(4):507-511.

Kahn C. EMS, first responders, and crash injury. *Top Emerg Med*. 2006;26:68-74.

Kupas D. Lights and Siren Use by Emergency Medical Services (EMS): Above All Do No Harm. U.S. Department of Transportation National Highway Safety Traffic Administration Office of Emergency Medical Services. Published May 2017. Accessed November 16, 2021. https://www.ems.gov/pdf/Lights_and _Sirens_Use_by_EMS_May_2017.pdf

Levick NR, Garigan M. A solution to head injury protection for emergency medical service providers. http://www.objectivesafety .net/LevickIEA2006.pdf

Lowrie J, Brownlow H. The impact of sleep deprivation and alcohol on driving: a comparative study. *BMC Public Health*. 2020;20(1). doi:10.1186/s12889-020-09095-5

Monoc's Siren Public Service Announcement. YouTube. Accessed April 6, 2021. https://www.youtube.com/watch?v=ivHTkZa7z0E

National Highway Traffic Safety Administration. Traffic Safety Facts 2018: A Compilation of Motor Vehicle Crash Data. 2020:92. Accessed March 16, 2021. https://crashstats.nhtsa. dot.gov

National Highway Traffic Safety Administration. Traffic Safety Facts. National Highway Traffic Safety Administration. Published October 2020. Accessed March 16, 2021. https:// crashstats.nhtsa.dot.gov/Api/Public/ViewPublication/813021

National Highway Traffic Safety Administration. *Working Group Best Practice Recommendations for the Safe Transportation of Children in Emergency Ground Ambulances*. Washington, DC: NHTSA; 2012.

National Institute for Occupational Safety and Health. Career fire fighter/emergency medical technician dies and paramedic is injured in a three-vehicle collision – Nebraska. Fire Fighter Fatality Investigation Report F2003-33. Published May 22, 2020. Accessed April 6, 2021. https://www.cdc.gov/niosh/fire /reports/face200333.html

Neo Film Reviews: MCL cinema Hong Kong Mobile phone car crash advertising effective. YouTube. Published June 29, 2014. Accessed April 6, 2021. https://www.youtube.com/watch?v =5Gtio4V1L3o

Olaveengen T, Wik L, Steen P. Quality of cardiopulmonary resuscitation before and during transport in out-of-hospital cardiac arrest. *Resuscitation*. 2008;76(2):185-190.

PRO EMS. Pro Policy 300.21 Driving standards. Accessed April 6, 2021. https://proems.com/policy-procedure-manual/300-operations/pro-ems-policy-300-21/

Safe Ambulances.org. Commission on Accreditation of Ambulance Services Ground Vehicle Standard (CAAS-GVS). Accessed October 13, 2021. https://www.safeambulances.org/organizations/caas-gvs/

Safe Ambulances.org. General Services Administration (GSA). Accessed April 7, 2021. https://www.safeambulances.org/organizations/gsa/

Smith N. A National Perspective on Ambulance Crashes and Safety: Guidance from the National Highway Traffic Safety Administration on Ambulance Safety for Patients and Providers. Accessed April 7, 2021. https://www.ems.gov/pdf/EMSWorldAmbulanceCrashArticlesSept2015.pdf

Turner DJ. RETT mobile and the future of EMS safety. *EMS World*. Published August 1, 2013. Accessed November 16, 2021. https://www.hmpgloballearningnetwork.com/site/emsworld/article/10978797/rettmobil-and-future-ems-safety

Wang H-C, Chiang W-C, Chen S-Y, et al. Video-recording and time-motion analyses of manual versus mechanical cardiopulmonary resuscitation during ambulance transport. *Resuscitation*. 2007;74(3):453-460.

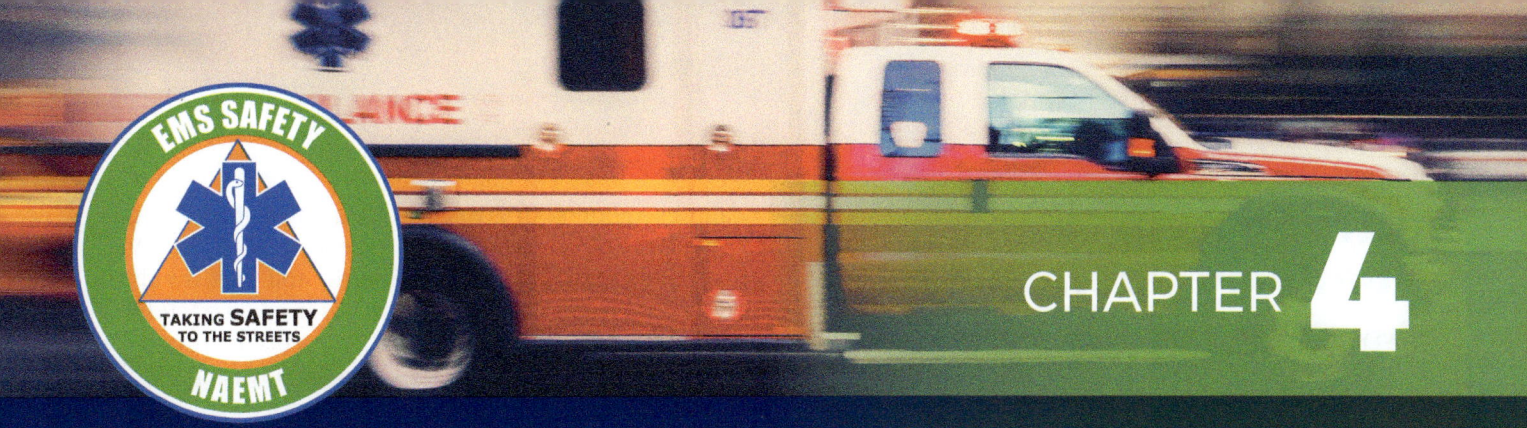

Safety in the Roadway

LESSON OBJECTIVES

- Identify EMS practitioner risks during roadway operations.
- Demonstrate the characteristics of effective roadway operations.
- Recognize the importance of a traffic incident management plan.
- Explain the concept of high visibility in roadway operations.
- Apply air medical safety techniques.

Scenario

It is a bright summer afternoon when you and your partner respond to a motor vehicle crash (MVC). As you arrive on scene, you find a downed motorcycle wedged underneath an SUV and a patient lying in the road. You park the ambulance as quickly as possible, and you and your partner walk quickly to tend to the victim. You reach the victim and find that his chest is not rising. After calling for additional assistance, you and your partner remove the helmet and begin ventilations. As you are getting your immobilization equipment in place and your partner continues to ventilate the patient with a bag-mask device, a car slides toward you. You yell a warning and leap out of the way. You hear a crash, and when you look up, you realize that the sedan missed your partner and the patient by about a foot before crashing into the SUV.

1. How should the ambulance be positioned at a motor vehicle crash?
2. What is your first priority at the scene?
3. What is your next action?

Introduction to Roadway Operations

Every day, emergency medical services (EMS) practitioners put themselves in harm's way when they respond to incidents on busy roads and highways throughout the country. While there to provide care for ill and injured patients, EMS practitioners too often become victims themselves when distracted or intoxicated drivers fail to see them and strike them with their vehicles. Roadway operations pose significant risks to EMS practitioners and other responders, as well as to patients and bystanders (**FIGURE 4-1**).

Over the years, both the federal government and individual states have enacted laws in an effort to curb injuries and death to emergency personnel responding to incidents on roadways. Currently all states have some type of "Move Over" law in place to protect emergency responders and highway workers. Additionally, national campaigns like "Move Over, America" have taken up the cause to try to educate drivers on actions to take when they approach emergency workers operating on a roadway. All areas of Canada, except Nunavut and Yukon, have a Move Over law.

Responding to roadway operations poses a significant safety risk to EMS practitioners, as well as patients and bystanders. In 2019, the National Highway Traffic Safety Administration (NHTSA) reported 41% of MVCs were due to driver recognition error and 33% involved decision errors. Recognition error is from distraction or lack of attention, and decision errors occur from poor driving. The National Safety Council (NSC) reports the following factors as being the highest associated with fatal crashes in the United States:

- Speed too fast or unsafe: 17.1%
- Failure to yield right-of-way: 7.3%
- Improper lane usage: 6.6%
- Careless driving: 6.5%

EMS practitioners should prevent becoming a statistic by taking proactive safety measures: before the incident, when arriving at incident, and when operating at the incident.

Not only are cultural changes needed for safe operations on the roadways, working together in our approach and management of roadway incidents is necessary to improve scene safety for all. This includes changing individual beliefs from "It can't happen to me" to "What can I do to prevent it from happening to me?" We need to develop an agency culture of safety in which all practitioners use safe operational practices during all roadway operations. We need to understand local protocols and response plans, use all available safety equipment, have the right attitude about safety, and work with other emergency response agencies so we know what resources will be available to us on the road.

Dangers of the Road

Over a 4-year span, 244 emergency responders were killed in the United States at roadside incidents. This included 192 law enforcement officers and 52 firefighters, EMTs, and paramedics. Roadside operations are a significant safety risk to EMS practitioners, as well as patients and bystanders. The statistics speak for themselves:

- According to the National Law Enforcement Officers Memorial, 12 law enforcement officers are killed after being struck by vehicles at roadside incidents annually.
- According to the National Fallen Firefighters Memorial, five fighters are killed while responding to roadside incidents annually.
- According to the International Towing and Recovery Hall of Fame and Museum, 60 tow operators are killed while responding to roadside incidents annually.

Unfortunately, there is no central point of data collection to determine the number of EMS practitioners killed while responding to roadside incidents.

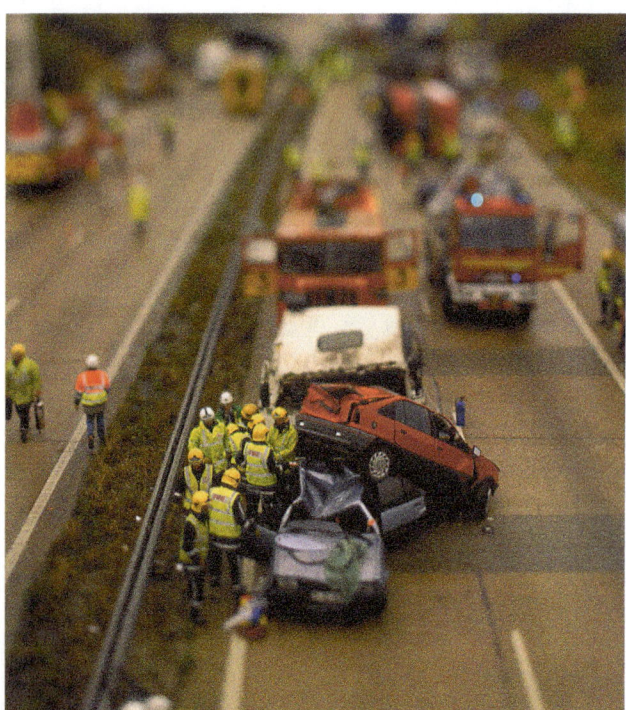

FIGURE 4-1 Roadway operations are a significant safety risk to EMS practitioners and other responders, as well as to patients and bystanders.

Additionally, finding the numbers of EMS practitioners who are injured is extremely difficult because in many cases, these numbers are not tracked. Add to this the number of near misses that are never reported, and you have a very large number of EMS practitioners who are killed, injured, or almost injured when responding to roadside incidents. Near miss is taught in aeromedical programs. Is it taught or even discussed in ground EMS education? For example: when taking a patient out of the ambulance, the person at the foot keeps walking, the person at the head lets go to shut the doors. The cot starts to roll but is caught and no adverse event occurred. Would this be reported as a near miss in your organization?

According to the NHTSA, on average, 10 crashes occur every minute that result in injuries in the United States. If we were to assume that each collision requires the response of two law enforcement officers, four fire-fighters, two EMS practitioners, and one tow truck operator, that puts nine emergency response personnel at the scene at each MVC. If we expand our view, we see the following:

- 90 emergency responders arriving at MVCs every minute
- 5,400 emergency responders working at MVCs every hour
- 130,000 emergency responders in a 24-hour period exposed to traffic hazards while working at an MVC

Because of the sheer volume of roadside incidents, it is critical that all emergency responders and EMS practitioners take proactive safety measures before the incident, when arriving at the incident, and when operating at the incident.

Preplanning for Safety

Work Zone Protection

EMS practitioners often respond and then must work on the roadway. This work zone should be protected, as much as possible, to limit the hazards to all responders and patients. What are your local standard operating procedures (SOPs; **FIGURE 4-2**)? What tools are used to stay safe and are those tools carried on each vehicle (i.e., cones, light sticks, flares, high-visibility apparel, etc.)? NFPA 1500.9.4 (2021) addresses the use of apparatus as a tool for scene protection.

When operating a roadway scene consider the following safety strategies:

- If using a fire apparatus, ensure that it is positioned at a 45-degree angle to the lanes (front wheels rotated away from the incident).

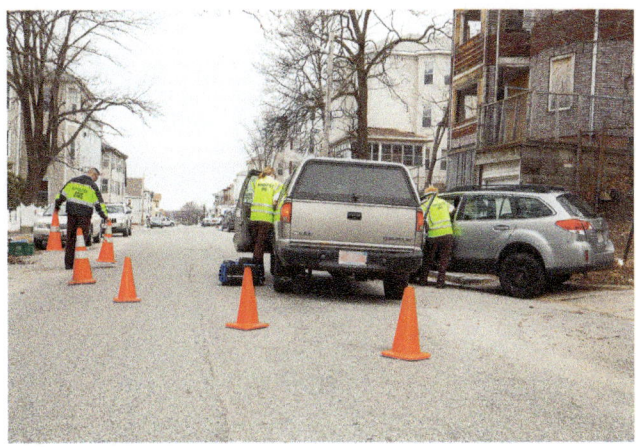

FIGURE 4-2 What techniques and procedures does your agency use to make the scene of a call safer?

© Jones & Bartlett Learning. Photographed by Darren Stahlman.

- If using the vehicle emergency lights when "blocking the right-of-way," differentiate between responding with emergency lights to "request the right-of-way" and setting up at a scene with emergency lights to "block the right-of-way." Multiple vehicles at a roadway incident with full emergency lights on can be blinding to drivers and decrease visualization of workers outside of vehicles.
- Extinguish forward-facing emergency vehicle lighting, especially on divided roadways.
- Reduce the use of lighting as much as possible at the scene.
- Wear appropriate highly reflective vests, day or night.

Stay in the Field

Before stepping out of the ambulance, ensure that no traffic is coming. Just as you use your mirrors when driving to ensure that it is safe to change lanes, check your mirrors and your blind spot to see if it is safe to exit the ambulance. If your view is still unclear, crack open the door to see if the path is clear. When you exit the ambulance, remember to stay close to it and keep your eyes on the road for any traffic. If crew members need to step down to exit the side or rear of the ambulance, they should try to maintain three points of contact when exiting the vehicle. Much like exiting a ladder, three points of contact are required (especially for larger vehicles): handrail, door, and step equals two hands and one foot, or three points.

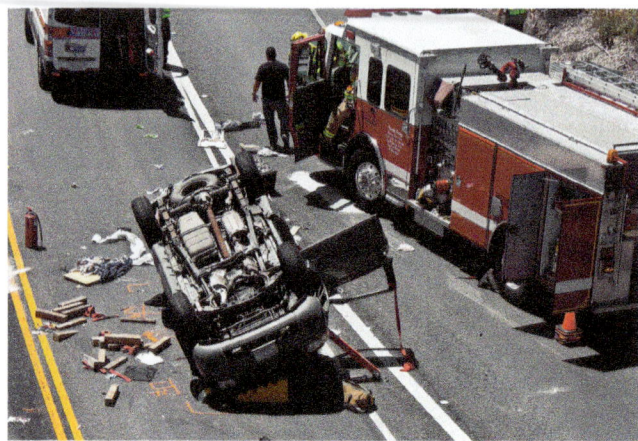

FIGURE 4-3 Fire apparatus should encircle the incident scene and block it off from all roadway traffic.

© pbk-pg/Shutterstock.

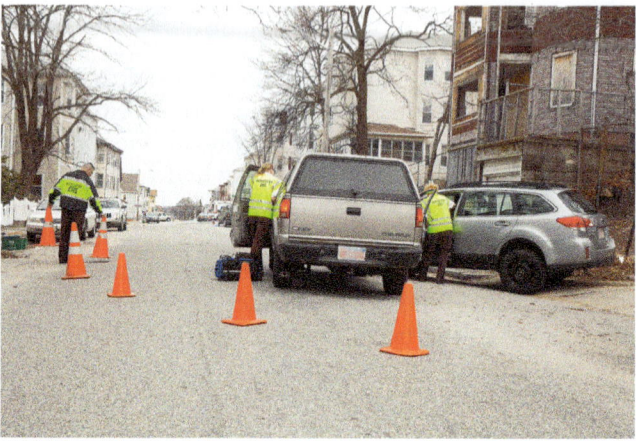

FIGURE 4-4 Line tapering can help protect responders from oncoming traffic.

© Jones & Bartlett Learning. Photographed by Darren Stahlman.

- Remain vigilant during all phases of roadway operations. Visually clear all directions before exiting vehicles. Never exit an ambulance from the rear compartment using the side door along active traffic lanes. In that case, use the back door and look out the window before opening the door.
- Maintain three points of contact when exiting the emergency vehicle.
- Have a multiagency approach to planning and operations.
- Get off the scene quickly to limit your exposure.

If your ambulance responds to a scene with law enforcement and fire apparatus already present, the fire apparatus should encircle the incident scene and block it off from all roadway traffic (**FIGURE 4-3**). If the incident command system has been activated, check with the incident commander on where to park the ambulance. Ambulances should park at a 45-degree angle in front of the vehicles involved in the incident. The wheels of the ambulance should be angled away from the incident scene. By angling the ambulance wheels away from the incident scene, if the ambulance is hit by a distracted driver, the ambulance will be pushed out into the roadway instead of into the incident scene and potentially those working there. The doors to the patient compartment should be facing the incident scene so the ambulance crew and the patient will be protected during loading procedures. After parking the ambulance, let any EMS practitioners riding in the patient compartment know which door to exit so they can avoid stepping into traffic.

Law enforcement should set up flares or traffic cones as line **tapering** to warn drivers that they are approaching emergency operations and should slow down and move over one lane (**FIGURE 4-4**). This will help give emergency responders the room to work

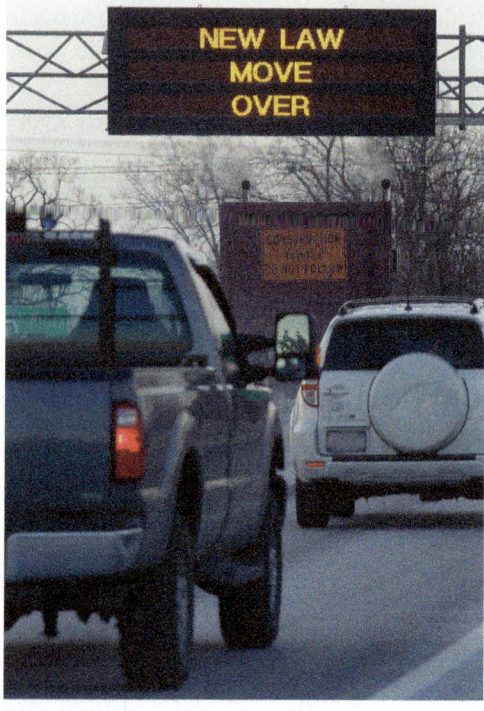

FIGURE 4-5 Electronic signs can warn drivers to move over a lane to give emergency responders the room to work safely.

© David Duprey/AP/AP Photo.

safely. In addition, law enforcement may close additional lanes, stop traffic, and even close access to sections of the road entirely. If the situation requires it, additional resources should be requested to implement traffic control measures that may include electronic signage (**FIGURE 4-5**). How law enforcement responds should be spelled out in the local traffic incident management plan.

Traffic Incident Management Plans

Because we cannot control every variable in every situation while operating on a roadway, every possible safety precaution must be taken to increase safety. To do this, every agency should have or participate in the creation of a **traffic incident management (TIM)** plan. A TIM plan is a prearranged and organized process that is undertaken to identify, respond to, and clear traffic incidents to reestablish the traffic flow quickly and safely. The plan will reduce the length of time spent on the scene and the impacts of traffic events. It will increase motorist, victim, and emergency responder safety. This is a document created with the input of all emergency responding agencies, from law enforcement, to fire, to EMS, to towing, and the Department of Transportation (DOT). A multiple agency response increases the number of "targets," and developing and following a TIM plan will reduce the time in which personnel are targets (**FIGURE 4-6**). A TIM plan ensures that all agencies will work together to secure the scene, maintain scene safety, care for and safely extract patients from the scene, and clear the scene as efficiently and safely as possible. The plan usually avoids having responding agencies depart the scene in a staggered fashion as this could lead to motorist confusion. Obviously, this component of the plan may not be applicable to ambulances as they depart when they have their patient loaded for transport.

In the Field

Traffic control is vital to the safety of emergency responders, patients, and bystanders and should always be rendered to the local law enforcement authority.

The TIM plan should spell out the roles and responsibilities of each agency, including arrival procedures, operating procedures, and how they communicate with their partner organizations (i.e., common frequencies, operating channels, and multiagency frequencies). The goal is that every agency and emergency responder will be operating in the spirit of interagency collaboration and with the safety of all emergency responders, patients, and bystanders in mind.

High-Visibility Apparel

Before exiting the vehicle, don high-visibility safety apparel. A typical EMS uniform is dark pants, dark shirt, and dark jacket. This ensemble does not do anything to enhance the visibility of the EMS practitioner. In 2008, federal regulation 23 CFR 634 went into effect, mandating that anyone working in the right-of-way of a federal aid highway must wear high-visibility clothing that meets the requirements of the American National Standards Institute (ANSI 207) and also addressed in NFPA 1500.9.4.9 (2021 version; **FIGURE 4-7**). This requirement applies to all emergency responders, including EMS practitioners, whether paid or volunteer. If you do not wear the proper apparel, in the event of an incident, neither you nor your family will receive any type of insurance, workers' compensation, or death benefits. Today, the high-visibility safety apparel worn most by EMS professionals is an ANSI-compliant safety vest because it can be worn over any garment at any time of the year, versus jackets that are typically only worn in cooler temperatures.

High-visibility safety vests and clothing must be worn in the day and at night. High-visibility vests have instantly recognizable fluorescent backgrounds and reflective strips. This personal protective safety clothing is intended to provide conspicuity during both daytime and nighttime usage and meets the performance class 2 or 3 requirements of American National Standards Institute (ANSI)/International Safety Equipment Association (ISEA) 207. High-visibility clothing, including the turnout gear for firefighters, includes reflective strips and trim. Most firefighter turnout gear does not meet this requirement; therefore, the responding firefighters

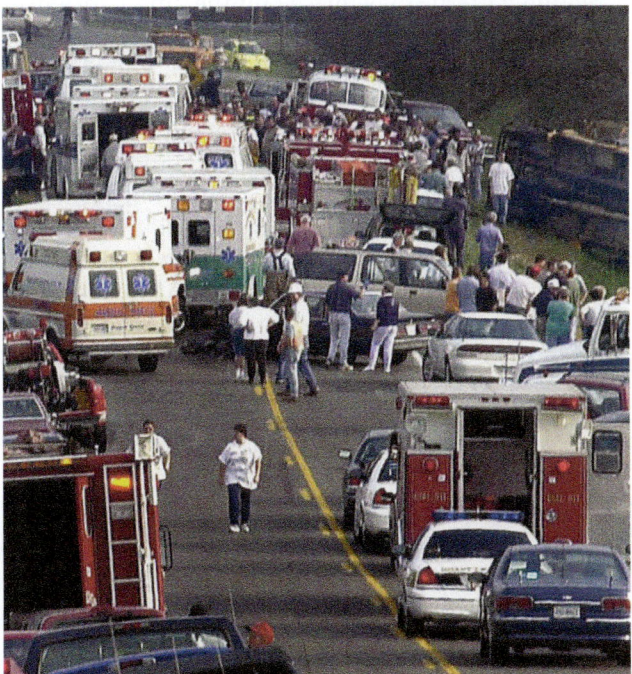

FIGURE 4-6 At a major motor vehicle crash, such as this one, traffic control can be very confusing without a plan.
© David Crigger/Bristol Herald Courier/AP Photo.

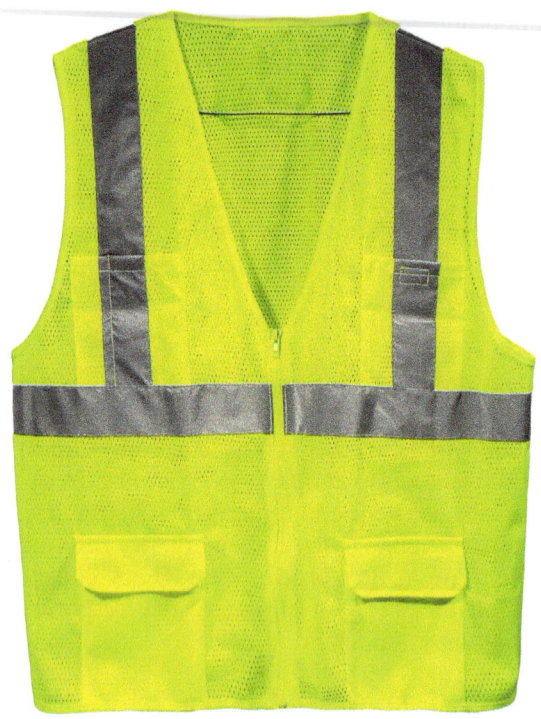

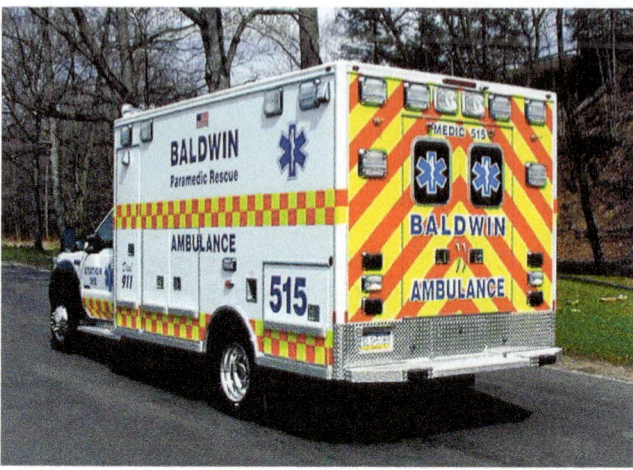

FIGURE 4-8 The United Kingdom has used the Battenburg pattern of alternating contrasting fluorescent colors (side of ambulance); it is also widely used in Europe. Chevrons (back of ambulance) are used in the United States because they are associated with danger or warning.

should still don high-visibility apparel (i.e., ANSI 207 breakaway vest) on top of their turnout gear.

Wear the vests when outside of a vehicle in a neighborhood and not just on the highways. Some agencies have a "boots on the ground, wear high-visibility vests" policy that requires EMS personnel to wear their high-visibility vests when exiting their vehicle on all responses.

Vehicle Visibility

Visibility of emergency vehicles is important to emergency responders, but even more important to the general public. You may think, "How can the public not see emergency vehicles when they are lit up like a Christmas tree?" In 2009, FEMA released a study, the Emergency Vehicle Visibility and Conspicuity Study (FA-323), on the importance of enhancing vehicle visibility using conspicuity products. **Conspicuity** is the ability of a vehicle to draw the attention of other drivers. Enhancing a vehicle's conspicuity is not just about making it easily visible but also about enhancing the safety of the emergency vehicle and the public. Various factors affect the visibility of an ambulance, including size, color scheme, and emergency lighting.

Studies have shown that flashing lights, versus steady, are far superior for gaining the attention of other drivers. A combination of red and yellow colors in the flashing lights package has proved to be popular

as a warning and caution identifier. The red and yellow are used because they signify "danger."

Research suggests that color, patterns, and reflectivity will make emergency vehicles more visible and help to reduce the incidence of other drivers crashing into ambulances. The use of contrasting fluorescent colors and reflective colors has been shown to assist drivers in locating hazards on the roadway, both day and night. Creating patterns to be placed on the ambulance using contrasting fluorescent colors increases the conspicuity of the vehicle. Since 2000, the United Kingdom and many parts of Europe have used the Battenburg pattern, alternating contrasting fluorescent colors, as the standard for its police vehicles and ambulances.

Because the Battenburg pattern is not recognized in the United States, researchers looked at the chevron pattern, which is generally thought to signal danger (**FIGURE 4-8**). According to NFPA 1901: Standard for Automotive Fire Apparatus, fire service vehicles purchased since 2009 have been required to have at least 50% of the rear vertical surface covered with the inverted V chevron pattern. The 2019 edition of NFPA 1917: Standard for Automotive Ambulances, requires ambulances to have at least the same pattern.

Retroreflective material offers another level of vehicle conspicuity. All too often, nighttime drivers have difficulty determining vehicle direction and motion. Outlining the contour edges of the emergency vehicle with retroreflective materials will improve drivers' ability to see EMS vehicles. Where chevrons are used, each stripe in the chevron should be a single color, alternating between two high-contrast colors. Combining all aspects of fluorescent colors, patterns, and reflectivity should provide a greater distance of visibility to other drivers and provide greater reaction time to avoid possible collisions with EMS vehicles on roadway scenes.

Vehicle Visibility: Using Your Lights

Use of your vehicle's lighting can be critical for blocking the right-of-way. However, it is important to avoid excessive use of high-intensity flashing lights as too many lights can increase the risk of emergency responders being hit (**FIGURE 4-9**).

Clear (white) lights should not be projected toward oncoming traffic to avoid blinding drivers. This includes the headlights of emergency vehicles. Be cognizant of the intensity of modern-day strobe lights and their effect on traffic approaching the scene from both directions. The flash of the lights, in conjunction with your reflective vest, could make you blend in with the light flashes.

If your ambulance is equipped with an Opticom device, it should be turned off. If the ambulance's Opticom is left on while parked at an intersection, it will continue to override the nearest intersection's traffic signal, causing increased traffic congestion.

In the Field

Responding to and operating at MVC scenes at night brings another set of hazards. It is human nature for drivers to take their eyes off the road and look toward the flashing lights. Drivers may also begin to steer toward the flashing lights that their eyes are focused on. This is called the "moth effect" and reinforces the importance of fire apparatus creating a protective barrier between the MVC and moving traffic.

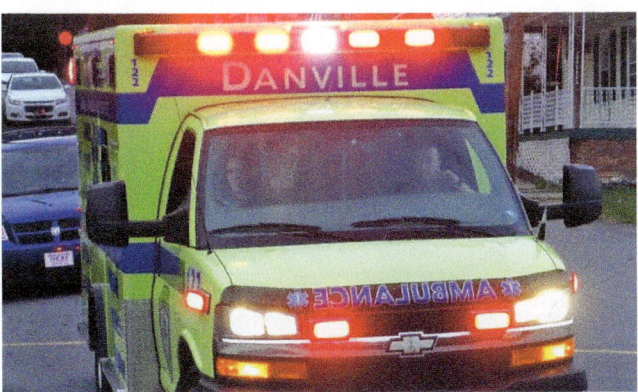

FIGURE 4-9 Be careful not to use too many high-intensity flashing lights at the scene as this can increase the danger to rescuers.

Courtesy of Douglas Kupas/NAEMT.

In the Field

One way to reduce the risks inherent to roadside operations is to limit the number of emergency practitioners responding to the incident. When conducting the scene size-up, you may determine that you do not need additional resources to safely manage the incident, and you may contact dispatch to notify them that no additional resources are required.

Air Ambulance Safety

The decision to use an air ambulance is determined by a number of factors, including patient status, the distance to the most appropriate facility, and protocol. If the decision to launch a helicopter is made, typically the incident commander will have his or her team set up a landing zone (LZ) near the incident, as appropriate for the surroundings and size of the incoming aircraft (**FIGURE 4-10**). Once on the ground, the EMS crew and

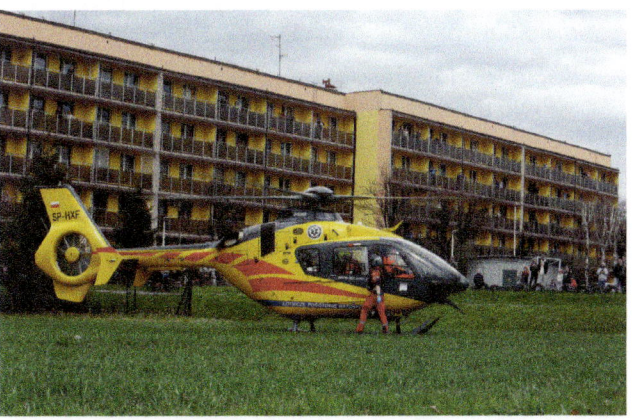

A

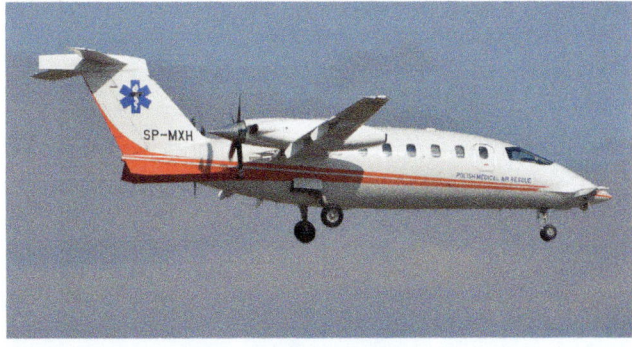

B

FIGURE 4-10 Be aware of the air ambulance services in your region. Examples of a medevac helicopter (rotor) **(A)** and a fixed-wing aircraft **(B)** are shown here.

A. © praszkiewicz/Shutterstock. B. © Przemyslaw Szablowski/Shutterstock.

flight crew will coordinate loading the patient into the aircraft using the flight crew litter.

Most aircraft will be on the ground "hot," or with the engine(s) on. Because of this, particular procedures must be followed when approaching the aircraft. Each aircraft is different, and the procedures will be spelled out by the air crew. Familiarize yourself with your local procedures for approaching and loading an air ambulance but always follow the direction of the flight crew.

In the Field

Your regional flight program should provide free LZ training classes for organizations. This is actually part of the TIMS "preplan" process. This requires an understanding of the flight crew and aircraft needs and an understanding of the final approach and takeoff (FATO) area (**FIGURE 4-11**). The LZ must be appropriate for the surroundings and the size of the incoming aircraft. Tips for consideration should include the following:

- A flat, level surface.

- Good solid surfaces where you can see any obstructions (i.e., low-cut grass, concrete, or asphalt).

- Avoid loose dirt or powdered snow that can get caught in air currents and completely obscure visibility impending landing.

- Avoid muddy areas of fresh cut fields as the grass will do the same as loose dirt and snow. The skids could get stuck in the mud and cause the aircraft to roll over on takeoff attempt.

- At least 100 ft. by 100 ft. form the LZ and add an additional 100 ft. by 100 ft. for each additional aircraft.

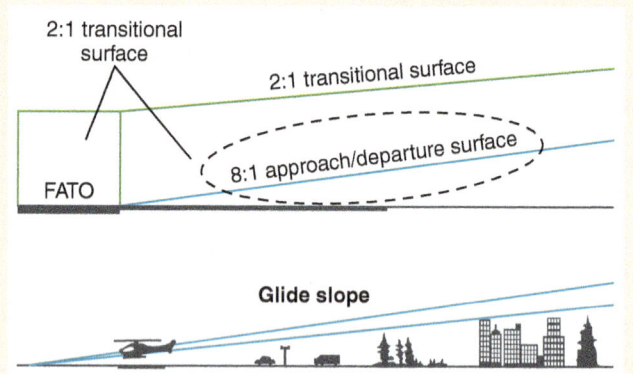

FIGURE 4-11 The final approach and take-off area for a helicopter.

- Clear the area approaching and departing to prevent straight up (maximum power) takeoffs. Think of an LZ as having a clear path to utilize like a runway if needed.

- If utilizing an active roadway try to utilize "hot operations" or relocate aircraft to an off-road LZ. You do not want the aircraft to have a mechanical issue while sitting on a major roadway.

CHAPTER WRAP-UP

- Roadway operations are a real safety threat.
- Traffic incident management plans are critical to reduce injuries and fatalities.
- Wear a high-visibility safety vest day and night.
- Use the appropriate number of lights with the right lighting during roadway operations.
- Communicate with air medical services to ensure safety for all.

SUMMARY

- EMS practitioners too often become victims themselves when distracted or intoxicated drivers fail to see them and strike them with their vehicles.

- Roadway operations pose significant risks to EMS practitioners and other responders, as well as to patients and bystanders.

- All emergency responders need to work together in our approach and management of roadway incidents to improve scene safety for all. This includes changing individual beliefs from "It can't happen to me" to "What can I do to prevent it from happening to me?"

- A traffic incident management (TIM) plan is a pre-planning document created with the input of all emergency responding agencies. A TIM plan ensures that all agencies will work together to secure the scene, maintain scene safety, care for and safely extract patients from the scene, and clear the scene as efficiently and safely as possible.

- In 2009, the Emergency Vehicle Visibility and Conspicuity Study (FA-323) discussed the importance of enhancing vehicle visibility using conspicuity products. Enhancing a vehicle's conspicuity is not just about making it easily visible but also about enhancing the safety of the ambulance.

- When responding to a roadway incident, you need to plan how you will help control the scene and help provide maximum protection to the emergency responders, patients, and bystanders. You must help control the environment in which you will operate.

- If your ambulance responds to a scene with law enforcement and fire apparatus already present, the fire apparatus should encircle the incident scene and block it off from all roadway traffic.

- If the incident command system has been activated, check with the incident commander on where to park the ambulance.

- Ambulances should park at a 45-degree angle in front of the vehicles involved in the incident.

- Before exiting the vehicle, don high-visibility safety apparel. High-visibility safety vests and clothing must be worn during the day and at night.

- Before stepping out of the ambulance, ensure that no traffic is coming.

- When you exit the ambulance, remember to stay close to it and keep your eyes on the road for any traffic.

- The goal of operations is to clear the scene as quickly as possible.

- Too much lighting can cause emergency responders to "get lost" in the scene clutter, increasing their risk of being hit by a vehicle. When possible, clear (white) lights should not be projected toward oncoming traffic to avoid blinding drivers.

- If the decision to launch an air ambulance is made, typically the incident commander will have his or her team set up a landing zone near the incident. Once on the ground, the EMS crew and flight crew will coordinate loading the patient into the aircraft using the flight crew litter.

- Familiarize yourself with your local procedures for approaching and loading an air ambulance.

GLOSSARY

conspicuity The ability of a vehicle to draw the attention of other drivers.

tapering A method to gradually direct traffic flow into an unaffected lane.

traffic incident management (TIM) plan A pre-planning document created with the input of all emergency responding agencies to ensure that all agencies will work together to secure the scene, maintain scene safety, care for and safely extract patients from the scene, and clear the scene as efficiently and safely as possible.

REFERENCES

American Automobile Association. Slow Down/Move Over. Accessed October 18, 2021. https://exchange.aaa.com/automotive/roadside-assistance/slow-down-move-over/

De Lorenzo R, Eilers M. Lights and sirens: a review of emergency vehicle warning systems. *Ann Emerg Med.* 1991;20(12):1331-1335.

Federal Aviation Administration. Advisory Circular: Heliport Design. Published April 24, 2012. Accessed March 17, 2021. https://www.faa.gov/documentLibrary/media/Advisory_Circular/150_5390_2c.pdf

Federal Emergency Management Association. *Emergency Vehicle Visibility and Conspicuity Study (FA-323).* Washington, DC: U.S. Department of Homeland Security; 2009.

Federal Highway Administration, Department of Transportation. Code of Federal Regulations: Part 634 – Worker Visibility. Accessed March 17, 2021. https://www.govinfo.gov/content/pkg /CFR-2009-title23-vol1/xml/CFR-2009-title23-vol1-part634.xml

Flannagan MJ, Blower DF, Devonshire JM. *Effects of Warning Lamp Color and Intensity on Driver Vision.* University of Michigan Transportation Research Institute; 2008.

National EMS Memorial Service. Honorees: Kevin M. Ritchie. Accessed March 17, 2021. http://www.national-ems-memorial. org/honorees/entry/9/148/?sort=6&dir=ASC&pagenum=46

National Fire Protection Association. NFPA 1500: Standard on Fire Department Occupational Safety, Health, and Wellness Program, 2021. March 15, 2021.

National Fire Protection Association. NFPA 1917: Standard for Automotive Ambulances. Published 2019. Accessed October 23, 2019. https://www.nfpa.org/codes-and-standards /all-codes-and-standards/list-of-codes-and-standards/detail? code=1917

National Highway Institute. *National Traffic Incident Management Responder Training Program: Train-the-Trainer Guide.* Washington, DC: National Highway Institute; 2013.

National Highway Traffic Safety Administration. *Traffic Safety Facts 2012: A Compilation of Motor Vehicle Crash Data from the Fatality Analysis Reporting System and the General Estimates System.* U.S. Department of Transportation. Washington, DC: National Highway Traffic Safety Administration; 2012.

National Safety Council. Injury Facts—Motor vehicle safety issues: improper driving reported in fatal crashes, 2019 [Table]. Published 2021. Accessed April 7, 2021. https:// injuryfacts.nsc.org/motor-vehicle/motor-vehicle-safety-issues /improper-driving-and-road-rage/

State of New Jersey. *New Jersey Highway Incident Traffic Safety Guidelines for Emergency Responders.* State of New Jersey; 2010.

U.S. Bureau of Labor Statistics. Fatal Occupational Injuries to Emergency Responders. Accessed April 7, 2021. https://www .bls.gov/iif/oshwc/cfoi/er_fact_sheet.htm

U.S. Fire Administration. Emergency Vehicle Safety Initiative. February, 2014. Accessed March 16, 2021. https://www.usfa .fema.gov/downloads/pdf/publications/fa_336.pdf

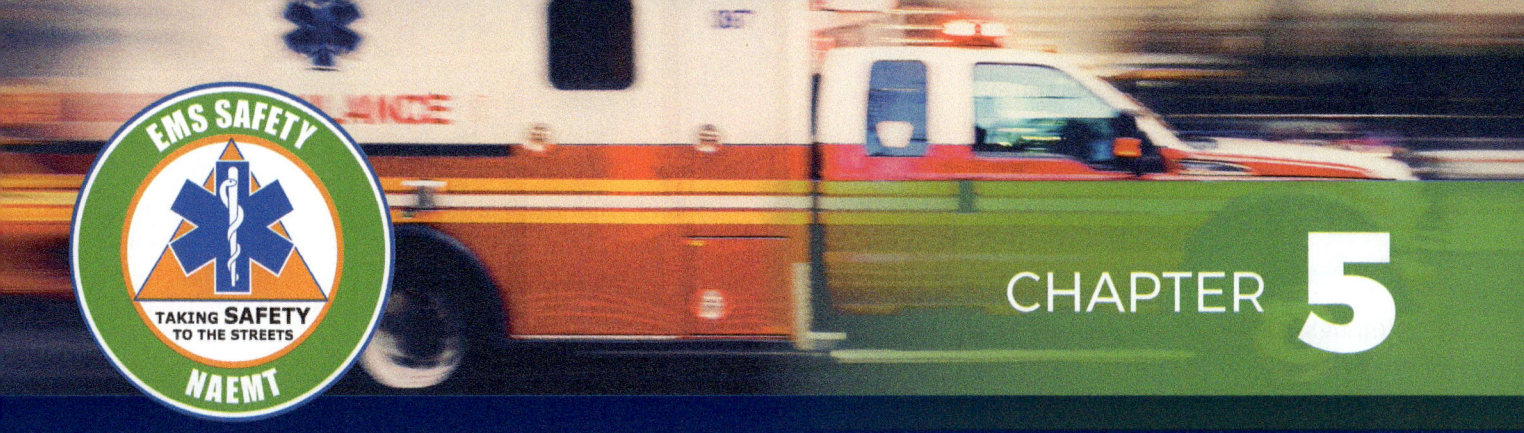

CHAPTER 5

Patient Safety

LESSON OBJECTIVES

- Describe how to mitigate errors in patient care.
- Identify patient safety events.
- Recognize the steps to improve patient safety reporting.

- Discuss unsafe conditions that could contribute to patient care errors and adverse events.
- Demonstrate safe and effective adult, pediatric, geriatric, and bariatric patient handling techniques.

Scenario

At the end of your 24-hour shift, you are dispatched to an extended care facility to transport a stretcher-bound patient to dialysis. You and your partner arrive to find the patient unresponsive. After obtaining the transfer report, you place the stack of paperwork under the patient's feet.

Your partner takes the position at the head of the stretcher, and you exit the facility with the patient. As you guide the stretcher down the bumpy sidewalk, you notice that the paperwork is flying away. Without speaking, you let go of the stretcher to chase down the paperwork. Your partner sees the paperwork out of the corner of her eye, and without speaking, she lets go of the stretcher to chase it down. The stretcher continues down the sidewalk and stops suddenly when the wheel hits a large bump. The stretcher tips over, and the patient remains attached to the stretcher. However, he bumps his head on the curb and sustains a serious head injury.

1. What errors were made?
2. What could have been done differently?
3. How does situational awareness apply here?

Introduction to Patient Safety

Although we would like to think otherwise, medical professionals, including emergency medical services (EMS) practitioners, are human and do make mistakes. EMS agencies must be cognizant of the fact that errors are inevitable. For this reason, we must strive to design EMS systems that minimize the risk to patients and EMS practitioners when providing care. Systems designed to eliminate all human error are doomed to fail, because making errors is part of a normal human process. Ideally, our systems should aim to limit preventable errors that occur due to lack of education or lack of proper resources (which present with their own limitations). The greatest benefit to patients is derived from systems designed with safeguards in place to "trap" errors before they result in a near-miss or actual harm to the patient or practitioner, or both (**FIGURE 5-1**). In this chapter, we discuss several areas that have been identified as being prone to error and discuss ways to minimize the risks and reduce errors. Later in this chapter we will discuss how patient errors most often occur and prevention methods to reduce errors.

Medical Error

According to the 1999 Institute of Medicine (IOM) report, *To Err is Human*, medical errors occur far too often among the healthcare practitioner population. Errors represent a deviation from a process that may or may not lead to harm in patients, using an incorrect plan to achieve an outcome, an error in the execution of care, and an unintended act. This report prompted the creation of the Healthcare Research and Quality Act of 1999. The report estimated 44,000 to 98,000 annual inpatient hospital deaths due to preventable medical errors. One study on prehospital intubations found that

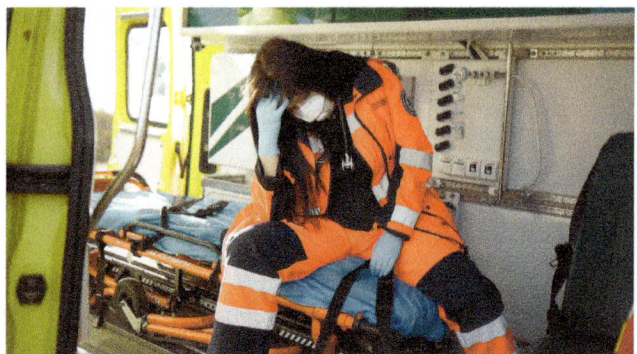

FIGURE 5-1 Human beings make mistakes. How we handle them and prevent future errors is important.
© dissx/Shutterstock.

25% of endotracheal tubes in the field are misplaced, with 67% of them being placed in the esophagus and 33% in the hypopharynx.

Since 1999, various studies have revealed even higher numbers of inpatient deaths due to preventable medical errors. Actually if "medical error" were listed on U.S. death statistics (which it currently is not), it would be the third leading cause of death in the country, only surpassed by heart disease and cancer. Some publications have attributed over 400,000 annual inpatient deaths as the result of preventable medical errors.

Error Types

Ways in which errors occur in patient care include the following types: (1) diagnostic errors, (2) treatment errors, (3) preventive errors, and (4) other error types. Specific examples could include the following:

- **Diagnostic errors.** Include errors in delay of diagnosis, failure to employ indicated test(s) such as a 12-lead ECG, use of outdated test(s) or therapy, and failure to act on results of monitoring or testing. An example could be a crew that does not employ the use of a 12-lead ECG for a patient with chest pain. As a result, the crew fails to realize that the patient is actually having an acute myocardial infarction and not just muscle strain, anxiety, or the flu.
- **Treatment errors.** Include errors in the performance of an operation, procedure, or test. Types of errors include: an error in administering care or in the dose or method of using a medication, an avoidable delay in treatment or responding to an abnormal test, and inappropriate or not indicated care. An example could be administering epinephrine to a pediatric patient, but the practitioner incorrectly calculates the dose (used 0.1 mg/kg instead of 0.01 mg/kg) and inadvertently administers a 10-fold overdose of medication to the patient.
- **Preventive errors.** Include the failure to provide prophylactic care to a patient or inadequate monitoring or follow-up of care. An example would be a paramedic who does not utilize continuous waveform capnography after intubating a patient. As a result, the healthcare practitioner fails to recognize an accidental extubation that occurs while loading the patient into the ambulance.
- **Other errors.** Include failure of communication, equipment failures, and other system failures. An example could include the crew members routinely failing to check their ambulance at the beginning of the shift because the off-going crew stated, "the truck is good to go." As a result, the on-coming crew fails to recognize that the 12-lead ECG cable

is missing from the cardiac monitor equipment. This lack of equipment is not recognized until they are with a patient who is complaining of chest pain, and now the crew has no ability to perform a 12-lead ECG.

Patient Safety Events

Patient safety events (PSEs) are not only classified by the error that caused the event, but also by the outcome of the error. Classifications of PSE outcomes include adverse events, sentinel events, no-harm events, near-miss events, and hazardous conditions. An **adverse event** is an event that resulted in harm to the patient. An example would be while a patient is being loaded into the ambulance the patient's right arm is caught between the stretcher rail and the wall of the ambulance, resulting in a laceration to the patient's arm. A **sentinel event** is considered a subcategory of adverse events and causes either death, permanent harm, or severe temporary harm. An example would be a crew walking to their ambulance with a patient and as they are approaching the ambulance the stretcher wheel is caught in a pothole and the stretcher and patient fall to the ground. The patient strikes their head on the pavement and is immediately rendered unconscious. The crew immediately transports the patient to a trauma center where the patient is diagnosed with an epidural hematoma. The patient ultimately recovers and regains full function, but due to the "severe temporary harm" caused this is ruled a sentinel event. A **no-harm event** is an error in patient care that does not result in harm. An example could be an incorrect medication dose administered to the patient but there is no harm caused to the patient. A **near-miss event** is an error in patient care that occurs but is caught before it reaches the patient. An example would be the wrong medication being drawn into a syringe, but the error is recognized prior to medication administration. A *hazardous condition* is a circumstance that increases the probability of an adverse event. An example would be two different medication vials that look similar being stored next to each other in a medication kit.

Unsafe Conditions and Acts

Many errors are made due to caregiver interactions with unsafe conditions. When unsafe conditions are combined with unsafe actions, such as complacency, the result is an error that could result in harm. Indeed, even if there was no unsafe action taken, the condition itself could still result in harm. Some examples of unsafe conditions could include (1) expired medications being carried, (2) improperly labeled supplies or equipment, (3) mechanical issues with transport

vehicles, and (4) mechanical issues with patient care equipment.

An unsafe action could result in harm even if an unsafe condition is not present. Commonly the result of complacency, unsafe actions also can be the result of malicious intent. Some examples of unsafe acts could include the following:

- Failing to perform medication cross-checks
- Not checking medications, medical supplies, and transport vehicles for deficiencies
- Taking shortcuts or being complacent
- Not following the protocols or standard operating procedures (SOPs)

Safety Reporting and Barriers to Reporting

Safety reporting is essential to evaluating the overall effectiveness of the program. Near-miss events are not unique to individual practitioners or patient care scenarios. Rather, common errors are made in each situation (i.e., medication dosing errors). Solving the predisposing conditions that contribute to errors eliminates the near-miss. Errors need to be reported to the agency leadership so they can be analyzed and measures taken to avoid them being made again in the future. Agencies may elect to allow for anonymous reporting of safety concerns (i.e., locked drop box) to avoid any pressure placed on practitioners out of fear of retribution from coworkers or management.

In a 2018 Canadian study, researchers surveyed over 1,000 primary care paramedics and advanced care paramedics in Ontario, Canada, regarding their perceptions on barriers to reporting patient care errors. They identified barriers to reporting errors as the fear of punishment by their organization and/or investigation by credentialing bodies. Many practitioners fear that unhealthy safety cultures within their organizations interfere with them voluntarily confessing to making a mistake that could or did result in patient harm because it would lead to punishment by the organization. Discipline could take the form of suspension, termination, alteration in shift structures/schedules, and reassignment to nonclinical tasks. As far as being investigated by credentialing bodies, practitioners are concerned that reported patient care errors could lead to investigations into their certification/license. The risk of decertification is a critical concern of losing one's own certification/license completely. Providers in the Canadian study identified additional barriers such as lack of information on how to report a patient safety incident and the extra time it takes to report a patient safety incident.

Steps to Improve Patient Safety Reporting

Efforts to improve patient safety through reporting errors and near-miss actions would include the following steps by your organization's leadership:

- **Eliminate the fear.** "Blame and shame" practices only incentivize hiding errors in patient care. When errors are not reported, the root causes that led to the error are not mitigated. The unresolved unsafe conditions can result in additional errors in patient care.
- **Reduce uncertainty and educate practitioners.** Educate practitioners on the process that will be used when an error is reported. This will reduce the fear of the unknown when an error is reported and also reassures practitioners that there is a structured process in place to handle these events. Educate practitioners on the importance of self-reporting patient safety incidents. Reporting near-misses, as well as actual adverse events, allows for identification of contributing factors. Elimination of contributing factors decreases the likelihood of similar errors in the future.
- **Increase accessibility.** Ensure reporting tools are always accessible to practitioners in a manner that is convenient and simple.
- **Develop better relationships.** Having mutual respect between EMS practitioners, medical directors, governing bodies (state, provincial, regional EMS boards), and hospitals can facilitate self-reporting of errors. Adversarial relationships will likely result in finding human error as the cause of a patient safety event instead of evaluating all of the potential root causes.
- **Provide feedback.** Ensure that feedback on reported incidents is timely, constructive, and meaningful.
- **Promote shared learning.** Share lessons learned throughout the organization to ensure that all practitioners can prevent similar errors. Use of real-life scenarios can improve quality of training and can reinforce just culture.

Just Culture

A just culture aims to create an environment/atmosphere of trust in which people are encouraged, and even rewarded, for providing essential safety-related information—but in which they are also clear about where the line must be drawn between acceptable and unacceptable behavior (**FIGURE 5-2**). When errors are not reported then there are missed opportunities for improvement. A just culture is not a "no-fault" system.

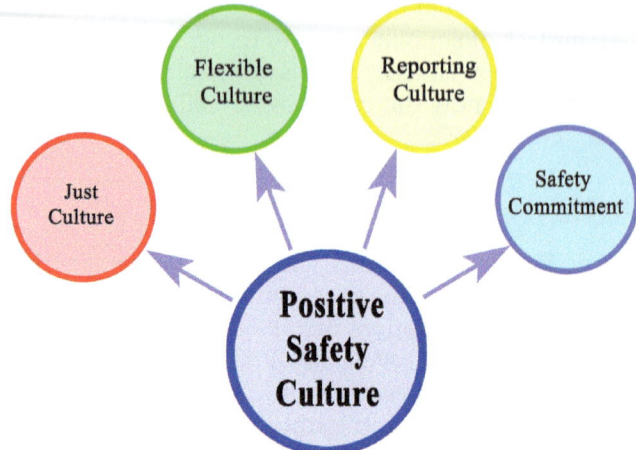

FIGURE 5-2 The relationship between a positive safety culture and just culture, flexible culture, reporting culture, and safety commitment.

© Dima/Alamy Stock Photo.

Rather, there is a difference between blameless human error, at-risk behavior, and reckless behavior. Human errors are expected and are coached. At-risk behavior is not tolerated but is coached and corrected. Reckless behavior is not tolerated, and corrective action is taken to ensure it does not happen again. These corrective actions can be disciplinary measures, such as suspension or termination/separation.

When an Error Is Made and Second Victim Syndrome

First and foremost, healthcare practitioners have the responsibility to report any errors to the patient's care team for appropriate interventions to be taken that will minimize the impact of the error. As an example, if you intended to give 1 mg of morphine but accidentally gave 10 mg, you have a responsibility to notify the receiving facility so they can monitor for signs of opiate overdose and can also avoid administering additional morphine under the incorrect assumption that the patient has only received 1 mg. Get a dose of Narcan ready and closely monitor vital signs, especially the respirations, in light of respiratory depression being an effect of the potential overdose. Ensure that information regarding the mistake is reported to your agency so corrective steps can be taken to ensure any system and human errors can be corrected. Near-misses are a warning sign of problems that could result in harm and should be treated the same as an error that caused harm.

Caregivers who commit an error in patient care tend to feel significant mental, physical, and social impacts as a result of the error. This phenomenon is called **second victim syndrome (SVS)** and can happen not only to the caregiver who committed the error but also to the other members on the crew. The stages of SVS that have been identified are as follows:

- Chaos and accident response: "How and why did this happen?"
- Intrusive reflections: "How did I miss this, and could this have been prevented?"
- Restoring personal integrity: "What will others think?" "Will I ever be trusted again?"
- Enduring the inquisition: "I might get fired!"
- Obtaining personal first aid: peer support and employee assistance program (EAP).
- Moving on: several scenarios are possible.
  - By dropping out, leaving the medical profession or moving to another place
  - By surviving and carrying on in the medical profession but with a significant emotional burden
  - By thriving with a positive take-away from the experience (i.e., personal and system improvement)

Recognizing practitioners at risk for SVS and taking appropriate action is imperative to ensure short- and long-term health for the healthcare practitioner.

Intubation Safety and Preventing Intubation Errors

Many advanced healthcare practitioners perform a low number of intubations annually. Knowing that, practitioners should use a structured approach to airway management that would lead to the reduced risk of harm to their patients. Studies report healthcare practitioners should perform 4 to 12 intubations annually to maintain competency in advanced airway management. Unfortunately, pediatric patients present an even greater degree of difficulty to field practitioners. One study reports successful placement of endotracheal (ET) tubes occurs in 48% of attempted intubations in patients. A 41% success rate was found in patients requiring multiple intubation attempts. Higher risk of mortality is linked to medical patients undergoing advanced airway management.

One study also stated that patients receiving basic airway assistance (e.g., oxygen with or without nasopharyngeal airway [NPA], bag-valve mask [BVM] with or without NPA, continuous positive airway pressure [CPAP]) had similar outcomes to patients receiving advanced intervention (e.g., ET intubation, supraglottic airway). The same study noted that patients receiving BVM ventilation (no NPA) were adequately oxygenated 90% of the time. Less than half of patients who underwent intubation attempts by EMS had properly placed ET tubes when they arrived at the hospital. Over

half of the patients who received prehospital intubation had ET tubes placed deeper than recommendations (Depth = ET tube size used $\times$ 3).

Preventing Intubation Errors

Having a structured approach to airway management can limit the chaos and confusion of a stressful situation as well as inform all team members of their roles and responsibilities and limit duplication of effort. The eight Ps of airway management is a good strategy for both adult and pediatric airway management and can be adapted based on local protocols. The following eight Ps approach should be considered:

- **Plan.** Plan for the procedure and evaluate your environment.
- **Preparation**. Position your patient appropriately and prepare all necessary equipment (i.e., primary airway and additional sizes +1 and −1 of primary airway size, rescue/supraglottic airway, laryngoscope handle and blades, ET tube introducer/gum elastic bougie, $ETCO_2$ waveform capnography, method to secure ET tube, monitoring equipment, BVM and suction, medications if drug-assisted intubation, oxygen, and personal protective equipment [PPE]).
- **Protect.** Ensure that patients who have traumatic injuries have in-line stabilization of their cervical spine.
- **Preoxygenation.** Avoid peri-intubation hypoxia. Use a nonrebreather mask or BVM ventilation prior to the airway attempt in order to limit hypoxia during the airway attempt. Consider apneic oxygenation via nasal cannula during the intubation attempt.
- **Pretreatment.** Some local protocols allow for lidocaine for increased intracranial pressure and/or atropine for pediatric patients. Always follow your local protocols.
- **Paralysis (if permitted).** Advanced care practitioners in some agencies (especially critical care transport [air/ground]) are permitted to perform rapid sequence intubation (or drug-assisted intubation), which commonly involves administration of medications that result in muscle paralysis. This is done to limit the risk of aspiration and to facilitate placement of an ET tube.
- **Placement with proof.** Intubation attempt with direct visualization and efforts to confirm placement immediately. Waveform capnography is the gold standard for ET tube confirmation. Other signs of proper placement can include visualization of chest rise and auscultation of lung sounds.
- **Post-intubation management.** Sedation post-intubation should be considered per your protocols. Avoid hypoxia, hypo- or hyperventilation, and utilize continuous $ETCO_2$ monitoring.

Medication Errors and Preventing Those Errors

The IOM report, discussed earlier in this chapter, went on to note that each year in the United States, an estimated 7,000 deaths occur because of medication errors. Studies report 1 in 30 patients are exposed to preventable medication harm in medical care, and that more than 25% of this harm is severe or life-threatening. Therefore, it is of utmost importance for EMS agencies and EMS practitioners to use strategies to help reduce and prevent these types of errors. These strategies include the following:

- **Double-check accuracy before administration.** Using a system to double-check for accuracy before administration of the medication is known to be a successful method for error prevention. One example is reviewing the "rights" of medication administration (i.e., right patient, right medication, right dose, right route, right time, and right documentation). Involving a second EMS practitioner in this process increases the chances of success.
- **Ensure competency with calculating dosages.** It is common for EMS practitioners to become complacent with their dosage calculation skills over time. Utilize pediatric emergency resuscitation tape or applications. Periodic revalidation of these skills is important for patient safety.
- **Seek uniformity of available supply for administering medications.** Although this is not always possible, it is beneficial to have uniformity in how medications are supplied. Consistency in concentrations, volumes, and packaging helps to prevent errors in the field.
- **Improve discrimination between medication packaging or spelling look-alikes.** Sometimes a medication has labeling that looks very similar to another medication. One way to help prevent choosing the wrong medication is to store the look-alike medications in different cabinets or drawers within the ambulance or in different sections of the response bag. If these medications absolutely must be stored in close proximity to each other, consider marking one of the boxes or vials with colored tape to distinguish it from the other medication.
- **Establish effective reporting systems that would encourage reporting.** Should a medication error occur despite efforts to prevent it, it is important that the environment within the organization encourage reporting. EMS practitioners need to know they can report errors to the hospital and their supervisors without fear of severe discipline. If EMS practitioners feel that their jobs may be in jeopardy, they will be much less likely to report errors, thus placing patients in potential danger. Underreporting of errors also inhibits an EMS agency's ability to discover and address any related problems within their system. EMS agencies that choose to promote a just culture within their agency maintain an environment that encourages reporting and supports the parties involved in these situations.
- **Pediatric dosing considerations.** Pediatric dosages for common medications can be difficult to remember because of the lower frequency of exposure to pediatric patients. Obtaining a proper weight for pediatric patients is critical to ensure they receive the accurate dose of medication needed. Job aids/tools are available such as length-based tapes and app-based software to assist healthcare practitioners calculating the appropriate dose to administer. Any job aids should be referenced with your local protocol or guidelines to ensure that medication doses are the same. Use of one of the commercially available resuscitation tapes assists EMS practitioners in determining the patient's weight based on length and provides the correct dosage for the most common medications administered in the field (**FIGURE 5-3**).

An alternate method to obtain a patient's weight involves asking the child's parent or caregiver the patient's weight. This method would be an estimate if the child was not recently weighed and should be confirmed with proper assessment of the patient. Some practitioners admit to not obtaining patient weights, rather they "just give a smaller, less effective dose." Failing to obtain an accurate weight on pediatric patients is hazardous and can result in over- or underdosing, leading to unwanted effects. A simulation-based

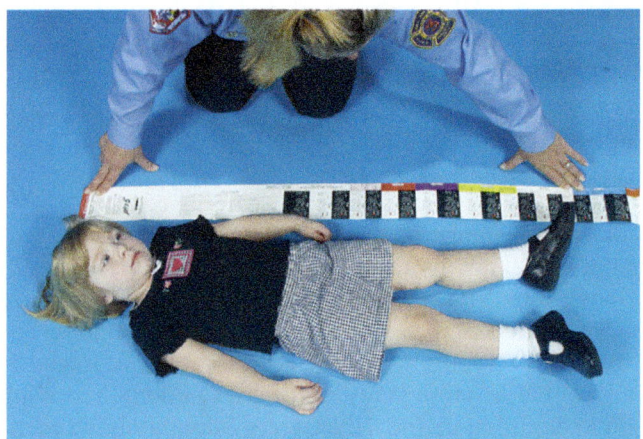

FIGURE 5-3 Use a pediatric resuscitation (length-based) tape to avoid errors in patient care.

study revealed that despite use of pediatric dosing references there was a 31% error rate in medication dosing in pediatric patients. This error rate was commonly attributed to the following:

- Failure to use the reference tool appropriately
- Improper dilution
- Air in the syringe
- Protocol errors

Finally, a study reports that the agency that developed the Medication Administration Cross-Check (MACC) procedure, as shown in (**FIGURE 5-4**), experienced a 49% decrease in medication-related errors after implementation over a 27-month time span. The most common medications administered in error were as follows:

- Ketorolac
- Lidocaine
- Magnesium sulfate
- Calcium chloride
- Lorazepam
- Midazolam
- Epinephrine 1 mg/mL

Deadly Shortcuts in Assessment or Treatment

EMS practitioners understand very well the importance of performing a thorough patient assessment in an attempt to discover the nature of their patient's illness or injury. If the physical examination of the patient is delayed or is less thorough than necessary, there may be a delay in the formation of a suitable treatment plan.

It is common policy to perform an appropriate patient assessment immediately after making contact with the patient. However, some EMS practitioners may elect not to follow policy on occasion, allowing distractions to interfere with their normal practice and delay the assessment process for certain patients. Some examples include system abusers, sometimes referred to as "frequent flyers," such as intoxicated patients and patients who appear to be suffering from mental illness. Often this approach does not lead to a negative outcome for the patient, which serves to reinforce the behavior. Repeatedly delaying the patient assessment or forgoing an appropriately detailed physical examination by taking shortcuts, only to find that it did not make a difference, can cause a shift in what is considered acceptable. This phenomenon is referred to as the "normalization of deviance" and can be very dangerous. As the "deviant behavior" becomes "normalized" and expected within the system, important assessment findings can be missed, potentially leading to negative outcomes for patients.

Equipment Failures

As with many professions, EMS requires its share of specialized equipment. For EMS practitioners to properly care for their patients, they must be able to rely on their equipment. When a critical piece of equipment fails, it can have a devastating impact on the patient's outcome. An EMS practitioner never wants to be treating a patient in cardiac arrest and find that the automated external defibrillator (AED) will not deliver a shock when the button is pushed.

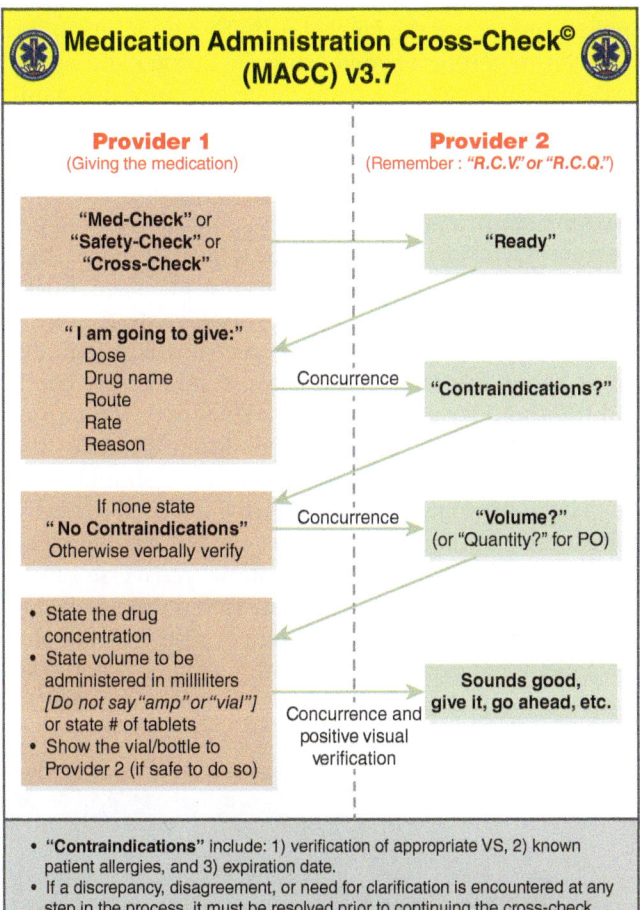

FIGURE 5-4 Use a system, such as the Medication Administration Cross-Check (MACC), to help eliminate potential errors.

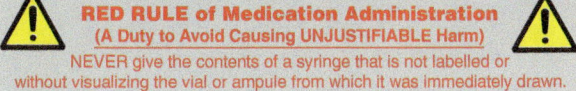

Stay in the Field

Depending on the patient care scenario, EMS practitioners may occasionally find themselves in a situation in which it appears that the best decision is to walk the patient to the stretcher. This situation must be approached cautiously because walking a patient to the stretcher poses inherent risks. Assuming that any increased risk to the patient's current health concern has been ruled out, the risk remains that the patient may fall by losing his or her balance, tripping over an object on the floor, or becoming tangled in wires or tubes to which he or she may be connected.

If the patient is to be walked to the stretcher, it is important to ensure that adequate staff are present to assist, the pathway is clear of equipment and other obstacles, and the stretcher is secured in position when the patient attempts to sit down. If the patient uses a cane or walker on a daily basis, this device should be given to the patient to walk to the stretcher. Although the patient is walking under his or her own power, the ambulance crew is responsible for the patient's safety. If your agency has a specific SOP on this issue, follow it!

Preventing equipment failures is a function of both the EMS agency and the individual EMS practitioner. Agency responsibilities include the following:

- Adhering to a preventive maintenance schedule that periodically verifies overall function, calibration, etc.
- Maintaining service records and failure logs
- Providing adequate backup devices to support the equipment, including batteries and adapters
- Maintaining an environment that encourages the reporting of equipment problems

EMS practitioner responsibilities include checking the equipment at the start of each shift—not simply that it is present, but that it works! Be sure to follow the proper procedures (i.e., battery rotation schedules, stretcher lubrication) as identified by your agency. Properly report any failures or concerns identified during your check. If possible, details should be provided regarding what occurred, when, and under what conditions. Maintaining functional knowledge of the equipment is also the EMS practitioner's responsibility. This is especially important if the equipment is used infrequently. By refreshing your knowledge and training, you will prevent operator error from being the cause of equipment failure. Prevention of equipment failure requires a partnership between the agency and EMS practitioners. Working together will reduce the risk of equipment failure and will help protect both the patient and EMS practitioners.

Adult Patient Handling

Patient handling is a critical component in all forms of medical transportation (**FIGURE 5-5**). Improper patient handling introduces an unacceptable level of risk for the patient and the EMS practitioner. It may also negate the effects of clinical interventions. For example, the rough handling of a splinted extremity will increase the patient's pain, thus negating one of the reasons that a splint is applied—to reduce the level of pain from an injury.

Even when performed properly, lifting exposes the EMS practitioner to the cumulative effects of mechanical stressors. Consequently, minimizing lifting is a goal for each patient movement event.

Always use all safety straps to secure adult patients to your stretcher. All safety restraints should be used per the manufacturer's guidelines. The straps should be snug and secure. The shoulder restraints must be used. Buckling all transverse straps and the shoulder straps on the stretcher is not enough. The correct position includes straps above the knees, at the waist, and at the chest, and the shoulder straps should fit snug over the tops of the shoulders. Shoulder straps should not fit across the neck or be secured without being over the shoulders.

Safety restraints are not effective if not used correctly. For example, if the shoulder straps are not secured effectively, the patient could slide out of the transverse straps, injuring the patient and any practitioner in the rear-facing seat of the ambulance. Use the patient restraints only for the patient and not for equipment during transport. Remember, complacency is dangerous and unacceptable.

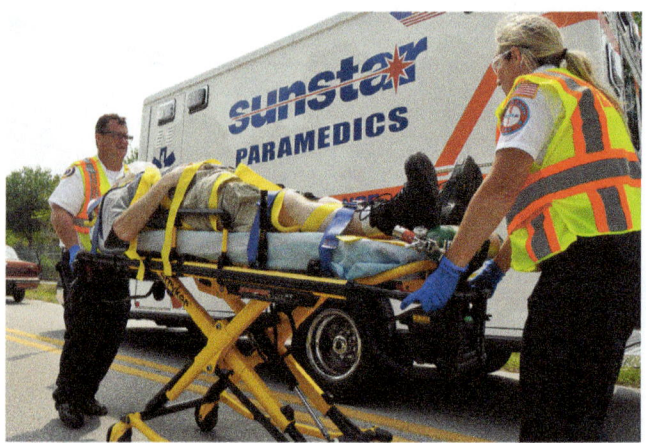

FIGURE 5-5 Patient handling is a critical component in all forms of medical transportation.
Courtesy of Sunstar Paramedics.

In the Field

Situational awareness is vital to safe stretcher operations.

Before moving the patient, you need to apply your critical thinking skills and anticipate everything that *could* happen during the move. Any potential hazards (e.g., icy sidewalk) need to be recognized and eliminated before the move.

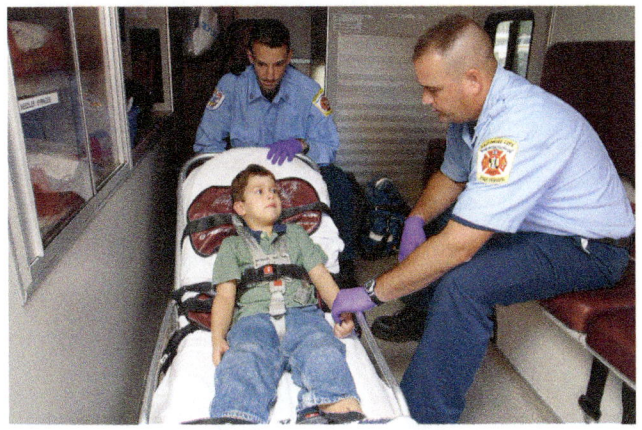

A

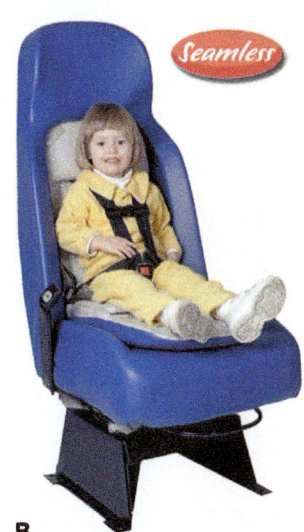

B

FIGURE 5-6 Pediatric patients need to be properly restrained on your stretcher before moving the ambulance.
A. © Jones & Bartlett Learning; B. Courtesy of EVS, Ltd.

Pediatric Patient Handling

Pediatric patients present a unique set of challenges to transport safely in an ambulance. In most patient populations, they are a distinct minority. Some EMS practitioners may not be entirely comfortable with pediatric-specific equipment because they have limited experience with it. Depending on the patient's age, children may be fearful of EMS practitioners. Communication could have a barrier, depending on the child's age, development, or primary language. Imagine a child trying to process all of the novel information that comes with an ambulance ride (**FIGURE 5-6**). If a child is frightened by an improper movement, will he or she be very likely to cooperate during clinical interventions?

The stretcher is designed for adults. Children come in all heights and weights, and they require additional child safety equipment that must be carried and used. We may not have the same comfort level with our pediatric skills. There is a natural tendency to remain physically close in order to comfort children, but this could lead to improperly restrained or unrestrained occupants. EMS practitioners cannot be complacent regarding using properly placed restraint devices designed for children.

Pediatric Patient Transport: Risk Mitigation

There are five situations in which a child is transported by EMS (**FIGURE 5-7**). These include the following:

- A child who is uninjured or not ill
- A child who is ill or injured and does not require continuous monitoring and/or interventions
- A child who requires continuous monitoring and/or interventions
- A child who requires spinal motion restriction and/or lying flat
- A child who requires transport as part of a multiple patient transport, such as a mass casualty incident (MCI) or newborn delivery

According to EMS for Children (EMSC) experts, *we should*: (1) Use properly sized child restraint devices, (2) fully secure child restraint systems per the manufacturer's guidelines, and (3) ensure *all* occupants are restrained when in motion. EMSC experts also agree *we should not*: (1) transport children who are not patients (alternate transportation in a passenger vehicle, when available, should be used) or (2) allow parents, caregivers, EMS practitioners, or other passengers to be unrestrained during transport.

A common misconception in EMS is that if a vehicle is involved in *any* collision, then the child safety seat is rendered unusable. This is simply not true! The child safety seat (**FIGURE 5-8**) can be used after a "minor" crash if *all* of the following apply:

- The vehicle can be driven from the scene.
- The door nearest the seat is undamaged.
- There are no injuries to any of the vehicle's occupants.
- There was no airbag deployment.
- There is no visible damage to the child safety seat.

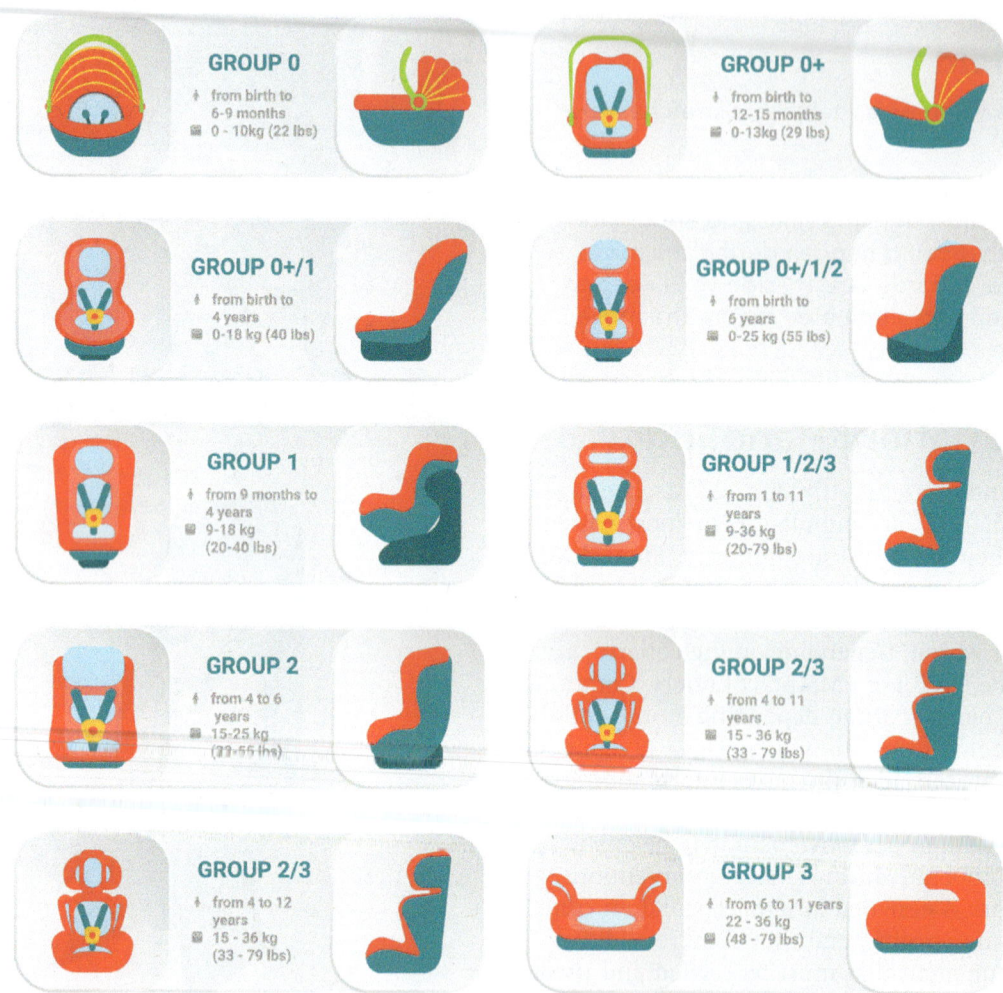

FIGURE 5-7 Pediatric patients not transported on a stretcher should be restrained in an appropriate safety seat.

© Garumna/Shutterstock.

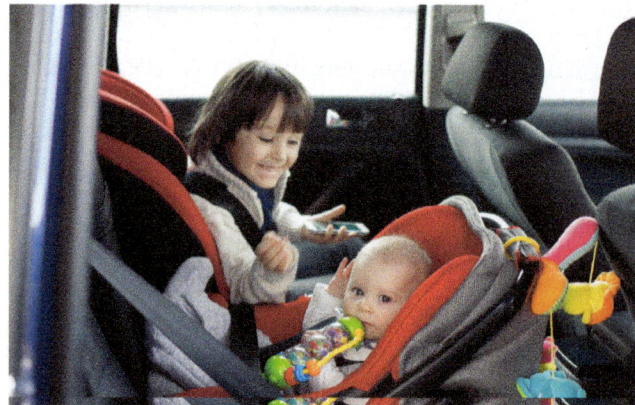

FIGURE 5-8 Child safety seats can potentially be used after a "minor" crash, depending on the circumstances.

© Tomsickova Tatyana/Shutterstock.

Naturally, if the vehicle is involved in a moderate or major collision then further use of the child safety seat is not appropriate. Another consideration prior to using the child safety seat is the patient's clinical status. Interventions such as immobilization or airway management will preclude the use of the child safety seat and will require other securement options.

Bariatric Patient Handling

Bariatric patients are more prevalent than ever. About 1 in 80 adult men weighs over 300 pounds, while 1 in 200 adult women is 300 pounds or heavier. Obesity increases the risk of injury to EMS practitioners and the patient. Part of caring for bariatric patients is protecting their dignity and treating them in a nonjudgmental fashion. In a society that aggressively values thinness, people who embody the opposite weight extreme may have psychological issues with self-esteem. With the weight of the general population on the increase, we need different tools for safe patient handling. Equipment can include things such as lateral transfer aids (e.g., slide boards, sheets, mattresses), bariatric-specific stretchers and/or seat belt extenders, lifts (air powered and hydraulic), and ramps or winches to prevent loading/unloading injuries. It may take more practitioners to safely move these patients. Any errors in movement may be more difficult to correct and may cause injury to the patient and the EMS practitioner. Ensure that the patient is adequately restrained while in transit. Failure to adequately secure the patient can result in patient and/or practitioner injury. The use of bariatric-specific stretchers and/or seat belt extenders could reduce injuries.

In the Field

Safe patient movement is critical for EMS practitioners because we have an obligation to our patients to "Primum, non nocere." This is loosely translated as "At first, do no harm." The literal translation is "At first, not to kill." Improper patient movement can kill patients. It does not take a dramatic stretcher (or cot, litter, or gurney) collapse or dropping someone down some stairs for a death to occur. Always keep in mind how fragile some of our patients are.

Geriatric Patient Handling

Geriatric patients may be impaired in the way that they process environmental cues. Common barriers to geriatric care include age-related deficits in vision, hearing, balance, and, in some cases, **proprioception**, or sense of orientation. Mobility is the most common disability and is reported in 1 out of 4 geriatric people

(**FIGURE 5-9**). This awkwardness creates an enhanced sensitivity to movement. Encourage patients to ambulate (depending on their clinical condition). Offer patients support by allowing them to hold your arm or shoulder to ambulate. Do not grab their arms or push them along. Move at their pace! Ask about hearing aids, glasses, assistive devices for mobility, and move them slowly. Because they may not be able to adequately process what they see, hear, or feel, geriatric patients may not be able to communicate their source of discomfort. Geriatric patients may process information more slowly, so we may need to alter the way we communicate with them. Explain what you are going to do before you do it, and explain what you want the geriatric patient to do, for example, "Please hold on tightly to this sheet and do not reach out, it may throw the stretcher off balance." It is not uncommon for geriatric patients to feel that they are losing control. Any clumsiness that we exhibit during routine movements will diminish their confidence in us, impair our ability to control the situation, and lessen the likelihood that we can implement safe lifting practices efficiently.

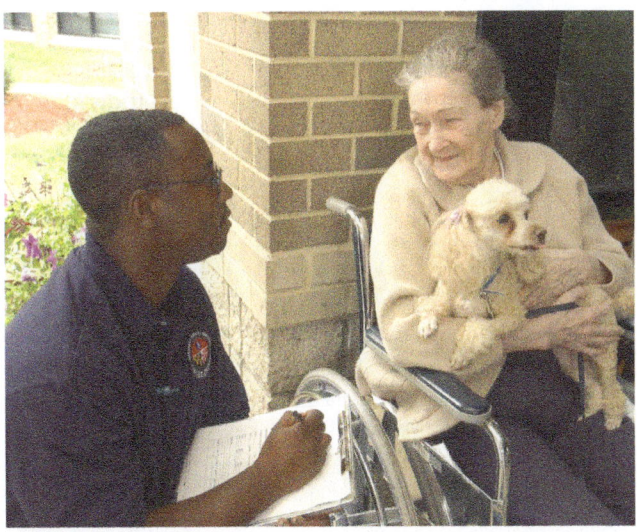

FIGURE 5-9 Geriatric patients often have barriers to care.
© Jones & Bartlett Learning.

CHAPTER WRAP-UP

- Making patient safety a high priority should be a goal for all practitioners.
- Identify barriers in patient safety and the steps to improve them.
- Near-misses are warning signs that should be taken seriously.
- Just culture aims to create an environment in which people feel empowered to report errors and adverse events.
- Complacency is dangerous and unacceptable.

SUMMARY

- Patient safety should be a high priority among all practitioners and their leadership.
- Medical errors present a significant risk to patient safety, and methods to prevent these errors need to become common practice.
- Both practitioners and their leadership share responsibility in identifying barriers in patient safety and the steps to improve them.
- Near-misses are a warning sign that should be taken seriously so we can learn from these events and not repeat them.
- Safe patient movement is critical for EMS practitioners because improper patient movement can kill patients.
- Specific safety concerns were reviewed for pediatric, bariatric, and geriatric patients.

GLOSSARY

adverse event An event that results in harm to a patient.

near-miss event An error in patient care that occurs but is caught before it reaches the patient.

no-harm event An error in patient care that does not result in harm.

proprioception The reception and processing of sensory information that allows an individual to have an awareness of body position.

second victim syndrome (SVS) When caregivers who commit an error in patient care feel significant mental, physical, and social impacts as a result of the error.

sentinel event A subcategory of adverse events that causes death, permanent harm, or severe temporary harm.

REFERENCES

Banja J. The normalization of deviance in healthcare delivery. *Bus Horiz.* 2010;53(2):139. doi:10.1016/j.bushor.2009.10.006

Carlson JN, Wang HE. Paramedic intubation: does practice make perfect? *Ann Emerg Med.* 2017 Sep;70(3):391-393.

Centers for Disease Control and Prevention. Prevalence of Disabilities and Health Care. Published November 26, 2018. Accessed November 16, 2021. https://www.cdc.gov/ncbddd/disabilityandhealth/features/kf-adult-prevalence-disabilities.html

Do it for Drew. YouTube. Published March 27, 2017. Accessed December 17, 2019. https://www.youtube.com/watch?v=239pVWepOHg

Dyson K, Bray JE, Smith K, et al. Paramedic intubation experience is associated with successful tube placement but not cardiac arrest survival. *Ann Emerg Med.* 2017 Sep;70(3):382-390.

Garza AG, Gratton MC, Coontz D, Noble E, Ma OJ. Effect of paramedic experience on orotracheal intubation success rates. *J Emerg Med.* 2003 Oct;25(3):251-256.

Gnugnoli DM, Singh A, Shafer K. EMS field intubation. In: StatPearls [Internet]. StatPearls Publishing; 2020. Updated November 20, 2020. Accessed November 16, 2021. https://www.ncbi.nlm.nih.gov/books/NBK538221/?report=classic

Hodkinson A, Tyler N, Ashcroft DM, et al. Preventable medication harm across health care settings: a systematic review and meta-analysis. *BMC Med.* 2020;18:313. https://doi.org/10.1186/s12916-020-01774-9

Hoyle JD, Crowe RP, Bentley MA, Beltran G, Fales W. Pediatric prehospital medication dosing errors: a national survey of paramedics. *Prehosp Emerg Care.* 2017;21(2):185-191. doi:10.1080/10903127.2016.1227001

Hoyle JD, Ekblad G, Hover T, et al. Dosing errors made by paramedics during pediatric patient simulations after implementation of a state-wide pediatric drug dosing reference. *Prehosp Emerg Care.* 2019;24(2):204-213. doi:10.1080/10903127.2019.1619002

Institute of Medicine Committee on Quality of Health Care in America, Kohn LT, Corrigan JM, Donaldson MS, eds. *To Err Is Human: Building a Safer Health System.* Washington, DC: National Academies Press; 2000.

Makary MA, Daniel M. Medical error-the third leading cause of death in the US. *BMJ (Online).* 2016;353. doi:10.1136/bmj.i2139

Misasi P, Braithwaite S. *Medication Administration Cross-Check (MACC).* Wichita, KS: Wichita-Sedgwick County EMS System; 2012. Accessed November 16, 2021. https://

kansasemstransition.files.wordpress.com/2012/08/macc-user-manual-v2-0.pdf

Misasi P, Keebler JR. Medication safety in emergency medical services: approaching an evidence-based method of verification to reduce errors. *Ther Adv Drug Saf.* 2019;10:2042098618821916. doi:10.1177/2042098618821916

National Highway Traffic Safety Administration. Car Seat Use After a Crash. Accessed October 13, 2021. https://www.nhtsa.gov/car-seat-use-after-crash

Ozeke O, Ozeke V, Coskun O, Budakoglu II. Second victims in health care: current perspectives. *Adv Med Educ Pract.* 2019;10:593-603. doi:10.2147/AMEP.S185912

Pepe PE, Copass MK, Joyce TH. Prehospital endotracheal intubation: rationale for training emergency medical personnel. *Ann Emerg Med.* 1985 Nov;14(11):1085-1092.

Reason JT. Engineering a safety culture. In: *Managing the Risks of Organizational Accidents* (p. 195). Routledge Taylor & Francis Group; 2016.

Sinclair JE, Austin MA, Bourque C, et al. Barriers to self-reporting patient safety incidents by paramedics: a mixed methods study. *Prehosp Emerg Care.* 2018;22(6): 762-772. doi:10.1080/10903127.2018.1469703

Studnek JR, Ferketich A, Crawford J. On the job illness and injury resulting in lost work time among a national cohort of emergency medical service professionals. *Am J Ind Med.* 2007;50(12):921-931.

The Joint Commission. Patient safety systems. In: *Comprehensive Accreditation Manual for Hospitals* (pp. 3-4). Joint Commission Resources; 2017.

Tweed J, George T, Greenwell C, Vinson L. Prehospital airway management examined at two pediatric emergency centers. *Prehosp Disaster Med.* 2018;33(5):532-538. doi:10.1017/S1049023X18000882

Wang HE, Balasubramani GK, Cook LJ, Lave JER, Yealy DM. Out-of-hospital endotracheal intubation experience and patient outcomes. *Ann Emerg Med.* 2010 Jun;55(6):527-537.

Wang HE, Lave JR, Sirio CA, Yealy DM. Paramedic intubation errors: isolated events or symptoms of larger problems? *Health Aff (Millwood).* 2006 Mar-Apr;25(2):501-509.

Practitioner Safety From Violence

LESSON OBJECTIVES

- Identify strategies to ensure practitioner safety.
- Demonstrate effective de-escalation techniques for a stressful or potentially violent patient encounter.
- Recognize the potential for violence against EMS practitioners.
- Discuss the safe application of physical and chemical interventions for agitated patients.
- Differentiate between abandoning a scene versus leaving for practitioner safety.

Scenario

At approximately 7:00 p.m., you and your partner respond to a report of a male in his 30s who is not breathing and has a weak pulse. On arrival, the patient's mother and a friend tell you they believe it's a possible overdose. You begin basic life support rescue breathing using a bag-valve mask as your partner prepares and then administers naloxone. The patient begins to breathe on his own and eventually wakes.

Immediately on waking, the person becomes irate and refuses further treatment. He stands, pushes you, and begins to verbally threaten you. You say, "At least let me bandage you up."

He responds with, "You touch me and I'll knock your teeth out!" as he raises his clenched fists. He then yells, "Get out of my house!"

1. Is this person still your patient?
2. Should you follow his orders to get out of his house?
3. Should you contact law enforcement and pursue criminal charges against this patient?

Introduction

Every emergency scene has the potential to create an unsafe environment for emergency medical services (EMS) practitioners. This is why the scene size-up is the first step of the patient assessment process. Some scenes may appear safe at first but then may escalate into an unsafe situation with few or subtle warning signs. Because of this, EMS practitioners must remember that scene size-up is a dynamic, evolving practice and they should never take anything for granted.

Every day across the country, EMS practitioners find themselves presented with potentially violent encounters with the patients they were dispatched to assist. Healthcare personnel account for 50% of all workplace assaults. In 2019, 67% of EMS practitioners in the United States reported being assaulted on the job. Approximately 2,000 U.S. EMS practitioners are seen annually in the emergency department (ED) due to assault. Injuries from assaults are higher for EMS practitioners than any other private-sector worker. These encounters place EMS practitioners, the patient, and even bystanders at risk. In a matter of seconds, EMS practitioners must decide if they should treat the individual as a patient in need of assistance or as an aggressive attacker. EMS practitioners must decide if they will flee the encounter or if they will stay and attempt to manage the patient. Managing this type of patient involves good communication skills and sometimes the need for physical restraints. When managing these situations, safety for everyone involved—including the patient—remains the highest priority.

In EMS you must prepare for a wide variety of calls. EMS practitioners train for low-frequency, high-acuity calls and practice those skills in case they are needed. However, little time is invested in training personnel on how to keep themselves safe against the increasing hazard of violence in EMS.

Illegal substances and a push toward increased outpatient management of patients with psychiatric issues have exposed EMS practitioners to patients who are experiencing delirium with agitated or combative behavior. A coordinated effort between law enforcement and EMS is required to handle these patients. Restraint of the patient is not always the answer, but in some cases, it may be the only answer. Later in this chapter, we discuss restraint concerns and techniques.

Personal Safety

As an EMS practitioner, if your overarching goal is to go home at the end of the workday, an awareness of safety should be a mantra that carries you through your day. EMS practitioners learn "BSI, Scene Safety" in school, although they rarely dive into what this really means. Safety should be a lifestyle, and it begins as soon as you commit yourself to a career in EMS. In the field, EMS practitioners should develop a sense of their surroundings to recognize and anticipate possible dangers. This sense of your surroundings is often referred to as situational awareness. When faced with a violent situation with a patient or an attacker, the EMS practitioner needs to quickly modify to a survivor mindset to maintain personal safety. Having heightened situational awareness allows the EMS practitioner to gain time when deciding how to respond in a violent situation. Situational awareness allows EMS practitioners to take in information, analyze the situation, and take appropriate actions.

At the onset of the response, consider the dispatch information, plan a safe response route, and follow local traffic laws. On arrival at a scene, be sure to stage the ambulance in a safe location, avoid blocking any other responding units or agencies, and take proper personal protection precautions. Ensure that you have a radio, that it works, and that the battery is fully charged. This radio may be your only way to call for help if necessary.

Secure Facilities

Examples of secure facilities include jails, prisons, and secure mental health facilities (**FIGURE 6-1**). EMS practitioners frequently transport patients to the ED for a psychiatric evaluation and may be called on later to transport a patient to a mental health care facility capable of providing short- and long-term care. There can be various levels of security within each type of facility.

In a police station or jail, initial care may be provided in a holding area or cell. Unless there is a mass-casualty incident or lockdown, correctional facilities prefer not to have EMS within the prisoner area and may transport the patient to the facility's medical center (**FIGURE 6-2**). Patients with behavioral or mental health concerns are sometimes outwardly violent to EMS practitioners, and practitioners should take appropriate precautions per local policies and procedures to prevent personal injury.

Stay in the Field

If your agency has a jail, detention center, or correctional facility within its coverage area, it is prudent to know your agency's standard operating procedures (SOPs) on how to respond to and operate within these facilities. If no such policy exists, agency heads should meet with site officials to develop policies. A preresponse plan is essential to ensure the safety of EMS practitioners. The level of response, placement of the ambulance on arrival, equipment you are permitted to bring into the facility, and how to safely access the patient are just a few of the procedures that should be agreed on by the EMS agency and facility staff.

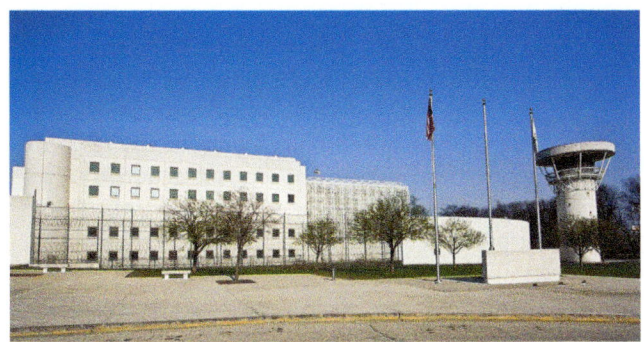

FIGURE 6-1 A prison is one type of secure facility.

© Benkrut/Dreamstime.com.

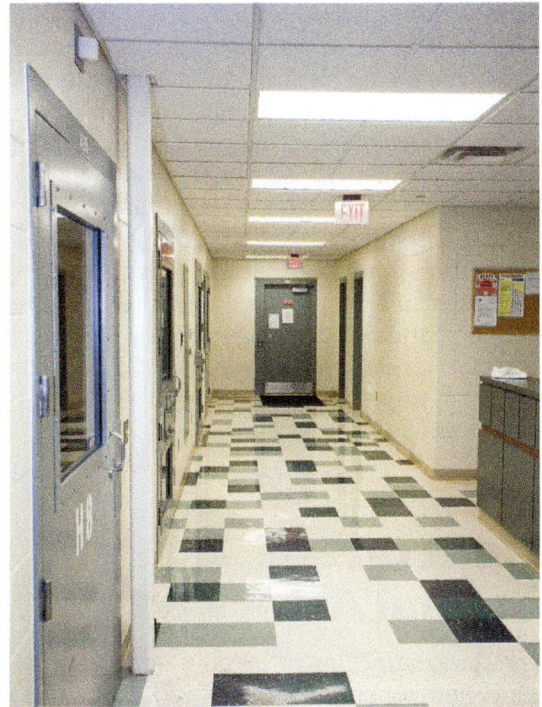

FIGURE 6-2 Correctional facilities will have transported the patient to the in-house medical center.

© Mikael Karlsson/Alamy Stock Photo.

EMS practitioners should be prepared for a delay in gaining access to the patient, as well as increased scene time because of security measures. Secure facilities will likely have a specified area for ambulance parking. Make sure you secure the ambulance on arrival. Travel through a secure facility should be only as directed and only occur with a facility escort. Wandering off could be dangerous and cause others to have to search for you. Remember, even though you are in charge of the patient's care, you are *not* in charge of the scene!

EMS practitioners risk serious injury if they wear a necktie. The tie can be used to physically manipulate the EMS practitioner and should not be worn. The same goes for a stethoscope, IDs on lanyards, or anything around the neck. These items can be used to strangle you. Common sense would dictate that weapons of any kind should not be brought into a secure facility—this includes handguns, knives/Leatherman, large flashlights, and full metal barrel–style ink pens. Trauma shears could be a potential weapon, so it is recommended that they be stored in the medical bag, under your control, and not openly visible.

The rules of response to secure facilities rarely change with the type of facility and must be followed to avoid personal injury or illness. Monitor the scene and your surroundings constantly. Situational awareness is important; pay attention if you suddenly feel uneasy or sense that something just does not feel right. Patients being transported from secure facilities will sometimes require a security presence on arrival at the hospital. Make this notification as early as possible so that security will be waiting for you when you arrive at the hospital.

Weapons

As the number of concealed carry permits increases across the country, the likelihood of EMS practitioners finding a weapon while caring for a patient is also increasing. Law enforcement officers and law-abiding citizens who are not affected by an illness or injury causing impairment to their mental state pose little risk. However, patients with an altered mental status who have a firearm can pose risk to the EMS practitioner.

EMS practitioners should have a basic understanding of weapons and how to safeguard them if discovered during a call or when having to treat a law enforcement officer. EMS agencies should have policies in place regarding the safeguarding of weapons in the field or on the ambulance.

EMS practitioners are not in the habit of "frisking" patients for weapons, but they should be looking for them during the physical examination and follow local policies on securing firearms. Patients who are conscious and legally carrying a weapon will most likely tell you that they are armed. Do not permit the patient to hand you a firearm. Even if you are familiar with firearms, do not attempt to unload a gun.

Patients with altered mental status who are armed and patients carrying illegal weapons pose a new and dangerous situation for EMS practitioners. Once a weapon is discovered, the EMS practitioner cannot just ignore it and continue with the assessment and treatment of the patient. If members of law enforcement are on scene, either you or your partner should inform them that a weapon has been found and allow them to secure it safely. If law enforcement is not on

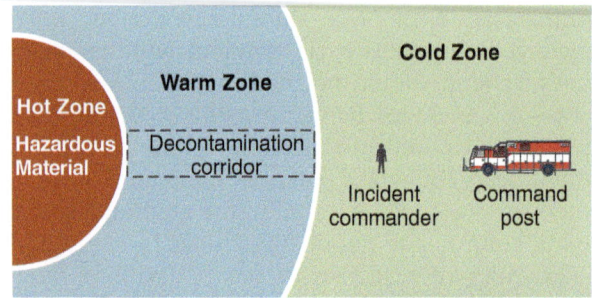

FIGURE 6-3 Safe staging zones.
© Jones & Bartlett Learning.

scene, follow your local policies, locate a safe means of exit, and contact law enforcement immediately. When treating an injured or ill law enforcement officer, EMS practitioners should allow another law enforcement officer to remove and secure any weapons. As always, follow your agency's training and SOPs.

Scene Hazards: Safe Staging

Zones of control should be established at every hazardous incident, and they include hot, warm, and cold zones (**FIGURE 6-3**). These zones, which are used at hazmat incidents, can be expanded as follows:

- **Hot zone/direct threat.** The incident area and the most dangerous area that must be restricted to essential personnel. Only specially trained EMS personnel are permitted in this zone.
- **Warm zone/indirect threat.** This area may contain a decontamination corridor if there is a potential for hazardous material exposure.
- **Cold zone/evacuation.** This is a safe perimeter area where EMS, nonessential personnel, media, and bystanders are located. This decreases interference with scene operations and helps to maintain safety. Vehicles, equipment, and additional personnel are also staged here.

The size and location of the zones depends on the specific incident. Preplanning and close coordination with law enforcement are keys to safely responding to violent incidents.

In the Field

EMS practitioners must realize that any type of response could be a potential crime scene. Crime scenes range from motor vehicle crashes to mass

murders and may include arson fires, domestic violence incidents, shootings, stabbings, or child abuse. The hazards at a crime scene may be physical, chemical, or biologic. All crime scenes have the potential to be dangerous, but active crime scenes have an increased risk, and EMS practitioners, unless members of a tactical EMS team, should not be anywhere near them.

Every active crime scene should have boundaries set up to protect EMS practitioners, patients, and bystanders. The boundaries are referred to as zones. The area where the actual incident is occurring is commonly called the hot zone and should be restricted to allow only essential personnel access because this is the area likely to be the most dangerous. The warm zone may contain a decontamination corridor if any hazardous material exposure due to a weapon is possible. Nonessential personnel, bystanders, EMS, and the media should be located in a perimeter zone, commonly called the cold zone, to ensure that incident actions are not interrupted and safety is maintained. Vehicle, equipment, and personnel staging will also be located in the cold zone. The sizes and locations of the zones depend on the incident type.

Patient or Potential Attacker?

The EMS practitioner must be able to distinguish between a patient whose mental status is altered because of a medical emergency and a potential attacker who may be under the influence of drugs or alcohol. When an EMS practitioner is not able to identify a potential attacker, the EMS practitioner may enter a potentially violent scene or remain in a potentially violent scene for too long. A person who verbally threatens or attempts to grab, strike, or spit on the EMS practitioner or who causes the EMS practitioner to feel apprehension or fear is a potential attacker.

Answering a few simple and quick questions will help the EMS practitioner determine if the patient is a potential attacker:

1. *Is this person trying to hurt you?* It seems like a simple question, but all too often EMS practitioners stay too close, too long with an aggressive attacker. Paying attention to "gut feelings" will help keep you safe by determining if it is time to leave the scene and call for law enforcement.

2. ***Is it this person's intent to do you harm?*** Is the patient's behavior intentional because of intoxication or irrational beliefs? If you think the person is confused due to a medical emergency, then the person is a patient.

3. ***What is your perception?*** Are you in fear for your safety? If you are, the person may be an attacker.

4. ***Why is the person threatening you?*** Is the person's confusion due to hypoglycemia or is it an act of aggression due to intoxication? If the person is confused because of a medical emergency, then the person is a patient.

5. ***Are the words backed up by actions?*** If a person is issuing verbal threats while holding a two-by-four, the potential for imminent violence is higher than if a prone patient is moaning a verbal threat.

In the Field

Responding to an incident during a civil disturbance may prove dangerous. To many, an EMS practitioner represents authority, and there is a possibility of being attacked by protestors. The mob mentality can cloud even a reasonable person's thought process. A police presence may escalate an incident, so EMS practitioners should load their patient as quickly as possible and leave the immediate area. Working in the back of an ambulance that is being rocked side to side by an unruly mob can be dangerous.

When dealing with a potential attacker, ensure that you have a clear path to exit the scene quickly and use your verbal communication skills to try to de-escalate the situation. Do not argue with the potential attacker, do not attempt to issue orders, and absolutely *do not* attempt to restrain the potential attacker. If you feel this person needs medical attention but is a threat to you, enlist law enforcement to secure the scene. The role of EMS is to provide care to patients and not to take custody of potential attackers. Follow your local protocols on care and transport in such situations. If your safety is in peril, leave the scene immediately and contact law enforcement.

Communication Skills During Times of Stress

To understand common signs of escalating anxiety, EMS practitioners must be aware of the powerful emotions present on many EMS scenes. How an EMS

practitioner handles these emotions can make the situation better or worse. Many of these emotions can be managed with good communication skills. Many patients (and their friends and family around them) are experiencing high levels of stress when they call. This stress is caused by anxiety due to the injury or illness and/or fear of the unknown. Usually when there is stress, the body will respond with some form of sympathetic response.

Look and listen for signs of anxiety or agitation in patients. Signs that emotions are high and an assault may take place include the following:

- **Speech.** Speech that is rapid and/or loud is common. A sarcastic and/or aggressive tone, possibly due to embarrassment, may be present.
- **Jaw or fist clenching.** This behavior indicates that the level of tension is high.
- **Fidgeting, deep or rapid breathing, and/or facial flushing.** These reactions indicate agitation.
- **Fixed, targeted stare.** This is sometimes called the "thousand-yard stare."

To effectively and safely communicate with patients, family members, and bystanders, EMS practitioners must develop a thorough understanding of verbal and nonverbal communication. How you say something, what you say, and how you look when you say it can affect how the patient responds to you and how much information you are able to elicit. "Do you want to go to the hospital?" or "Do you want to go by ambulance?" versus saying "Which hospital would you like to go to today?" may produce a different response from your patient. Based on your choice of words and tone and inflection points, you can convey very different messages.

Imagine for a moment that you are the patient. EMS arrives, and the EMS practitioner begrudgingly enters the scene. He throws his bag on the ground, and, with a heavy sigh while placing his hands in his pockets, he asks why you called for the ambulance. Do you trust this EMS practitioner? Did his attitude make you angry? Do you want to call 911 back and request a different ambulance?

There are already many communication barriers that you cannot control, such as differences in age, culture, language, and sensory loss in the patient; EMS practitioners do not need to build any additional barriers. Good communication skills build trust between the patient and EMS practitioners, and they help to offset the powerful emotions often present at incident scenes, making assessment and care easier and safer. Practice active listening, such as paraphrasing back to the person what was said. If someone is yelling, determine if that yelling is intended to be threatening or just venting. If the patient is venting, let them. If the patient is threatening, move to a safe area. While under acute stress, a person yelling about a situation is understandable and acceptable. However, a threat of violence made to an EMS practitioner must be taken seriously.

Poor communication may compromise patient care and put EMS practitioners at risk. Remember, you only get one chance to make a good first impression; solid communication skills will help to ensure it is a good one!

Nonverbal Communication

Nonverbal communication is also a large part of how you communicate with others. The position or stance you take, your body movements, your tone of voice, your facial expressions, and whether you maintain eye contact are all aspects of nonverbal communication (**FIGURE 6-4**). Words alone do not do the job—your body must say the same thing the words do. Maintain eye contact, without staring, when you are being spoken to. Maintain open-body positioning, because crossing your arms over your body could appear threatening. An open-body position without arms crossed conveys that you are listening. Consider sitting down and listening, if possible, because being on the same level as someone demonstrates a less threatening stance and can help people feel comfortable. Sit beside and face the person with whom you are communicating, as sitting across from someone may make them feel as though they are being interviewed or questioned. Sitting beside a person will allow the conversation to feel nonconfrontational. Do not fidget or play with

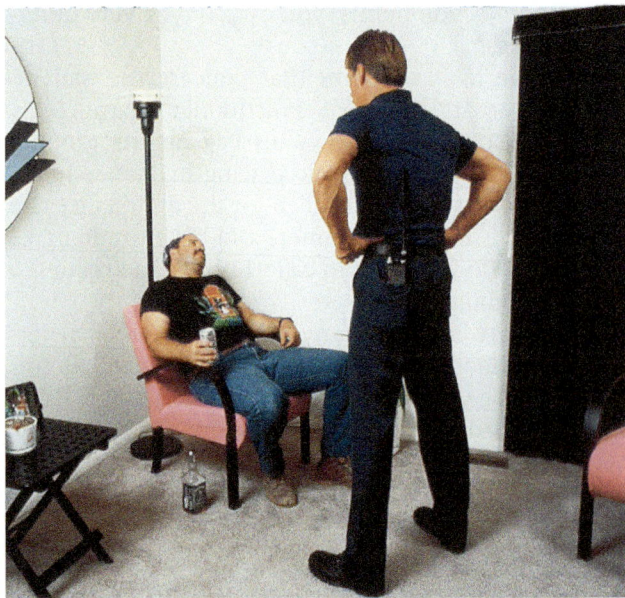

FIGURE 6-4 Your body language may transmit a completely different message than your words.

objects, such as clicking a pen, as this is distracting to the person who is talking. The fidgeting also makes you appear nervous or uncomfortable with the situation. These nonverbal behaviors can improve your communication skills. In many cases, it's not about what you say, but what you are doing. Effective listening shows support for your patient and their needs.

Communication works two ways. EMS practitioners must learn not only to communicate effectively but also to "read" the patient and bystanders around them. Illness and injury can create anxiety and stress, causing a person to act abnormally, responding with a sympathetic "fight-or-flight" response. This can occur at any time during the call. EMS practitioners can prevent possible assaults by being aware of the signs of anxiety or agitation, some of which are increases in the volume of speech, sarcastic or aggressive responses to questions, jaw or fist clenching, fidgeting, fast breathing, and fixed stares. Any action that gives you chills or makes you uneasy should be assessed for possible aggression.

Verbal Deflection and De-escalation

Acute stress reactions may manifest in yelling. Determine if yelling is threatening or venting. If the patient (or family or bystanders) is venting, allow them to vent. If the patient is threatening, *move to a safe area*. While under acute stress, a person yelling about a situation is understandable and acceptable. However, a threat of violence made to an EMS practitioner must be taken seriously! Verbal threats against EMS practitioners are often a precursor to physical violence.

In situations in which the scene is safe and aggression is present or anticipated, EMS practitioners can utilize verbal deflection, sometimes referred to as verbal judo, to diffuse the situation. Verbal deflection includes carefully choosing your words, avoiding sarcasm and judgment, neutralizing insults by responding with compliments, and redirecting the conversation. Often verbal aggression can be redirected by explaining everything that you are doing and involving the person in a patient care aspect; making the person a part of the care plan may put them at ease.

When practicing verbal deflection and de-escalation, EMS practitioners should adopt the **surveying stance** (**FIGURE 6-5**). The EMS practitioner's body should be slightly at an angle, with the hands above the waist and out of the pockets. The arms should not be crossed or fingers interlaced. The knees should be slightly bent with the weight on the balls of the feet. This is a neutral pose that shows respect to the patient. Maintain eye contact with the patient unless there is a known cultural difference that would require otherwise.

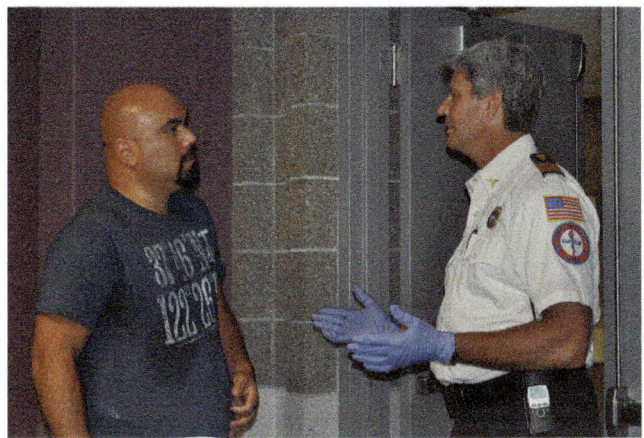

FIGURE 6-5 When practicing verbal deflection and de-escalation, EMS practitioners should adopt the surveying stance.

Courtesy of Sunstar Paramedics.

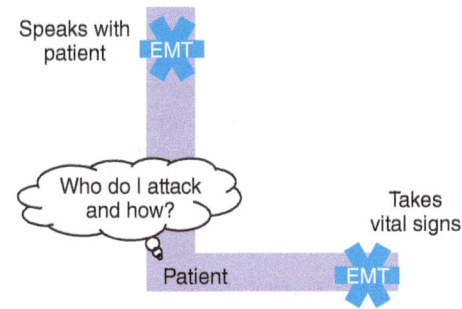

FIGURE 6-6 The assessment "L" formation.

© Jones & Bartlett Learning.

In addition to adopting the surveying stance, EMS practitioners should position themselves in an "L" formation around the patient (**FIGURE 6-6**). This is referred to as the **assessment "L" formation**. This positioning permits one EMS practitioner to address the patient from the front and one EMS practitioner to remain at the patient's side, taking vital signs and performing procedures. The assessment "L" formation gives the patient the illusion of personal space while remaining close enough to maintain a dialogue. The assessment "L" also creates a dilemma in the potentially violent patient—whom and how might the patient attack? If the patient attacks, this formation provides the second EMS practitioner enough time to escape and call for help.

If a patient attacks, EMS practitioners should yell loud verbal commands like "Stop!" or "Get back!" Yelling will alert bystanders that help is required and will get their attention. Always speak and act as if you are being recorded or filmed. Today, many people automatically record events on their cell phones and the footage may end up on social media.

Concealment Versus Cover

When sizing up the scene, maintaining situational awareness, you should make it your practice to always consider potential cover or concealment options should the scene rapidly change. **Concealment** hides you from view but does not protect you from projectiles or a potential attacker rushing toward you. Examples of concealment would include a bush, vehicle door, or shadow. **Cover** hides and protects you. Examples of cover include a wall, a thick tree, telephone pole, and the wheel or engine block of a vehicle.

Defensive Stance

If an EMS practitioner is met with a violent situation without warning and is unable to rapidly retreat, the EMS practitioner should assume a **defensive stance**. When threatened, the EMS practitioner should do their best to create a nonthreatening, nonaggressive appearance. Standing with hands up, with palms forward in an open position, keeping the elbows in, and angling the body 45 degrees to the patient is one option (**FIGURE 6-7**).

The AEIOU TIPS

As with any altered mental status patient, EMS personnel should consider all possible reasons for the altered mental status, especially when attempting to determine if the person is a patient or an attacker. The mnemonic "AEIOU-TIPS" is often used in training programs to indicate possible causes for altered mental status and stands for the following:

- Alcohol/acidosis
- Epilepsy

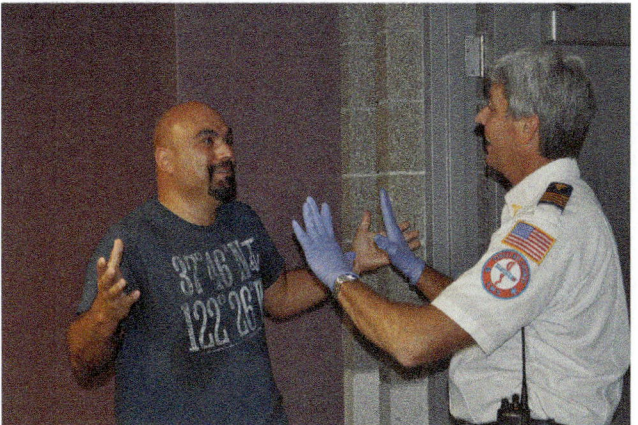

FIGURE 6-7 To assume the defensive stance, stand with hands up and palms forward in an open position, keep your elbows in, and angle your body 45 degrees to the patient.

Courtesy of Sunstar Paramedics.

- Insulin
- Overdose
- Uremia
- Trauma
- Infection
- Psychosis
- Stroke

Likely Scenes for Violence: The Six Ds

Likely scenes for violence include those involving the six Ds. Keep in mind that the terms in this mnemonic are only used in this memory tool; these are not diagnostic terms. The six Ds are as follows:

- **Drunk.** It only takes a small amount of alcohol to impair a person's judgment. Larger amounts can lead a patient to become intoxicated and commit uncharacteristic acts of violence. There is a lack of hesitation between the decision-making process and action phase. If it is safe to do so, assess the patient to determine if intoxication and not an underlying medical condition, such as hyperglycemia, is the cause of the patient's altered mental status.
- **Drugged.** The patient under the influence of illegal drugs or overuse of prescribed medications is a serious safety concern for EMS practitioners. Today, EMS practitioners may encounter patients experiencing unpredictable psychological responses like extreme anxiety, paranoia, or hallucinations from ingestion of illegal substances ranging from methamphetamine, to bath salts, to phencyclidine (PCP) or from overuse of prescribed medications such as oxycodone or fentanyl. Follow local protocols when interacting with patients who may be impaired due to substance use.
- **Diabetic.** When a patient with diabetes becomes hypoglycemic, very often EMS is called. Without adequate levels of glucose, the brain does not function well, and the patient may even appear to be intoxicated. The patient with hypoglycemia may become violent toward those nearby, including EMS practitioners. Take appropriate safety precautions and treat the patient as per local protocols.
- **Deranged.** With a patient experiencing a severe emotional crisis or a psychotic break from reality, safety should be the utmost priority. Carefully observe your surroundings, be especially aware of alternate means of egress, and never put the patient between you and a way out. Keep an observant eye for any weapons or anything that may be used as a weapon. Rule out the possibility of a medical condition as the cause of the patient's behavior. If

a behavioral or psychiatric condition is the cause of the patient's extreme responses, your communication skills are critical. Calmly convey the message that you are there to help and not judge or hurt the patient in any way. The louder the patient speaks, the lower your voice should become. Do not tell the patient to calm down; it might only cause more agitation. Follow your local protocols and contact law enforcement if you feel that your safety or the safety of others is at risk.

- **Domestic.** Due to more state laws requiring the arrest of the primary aggressor, a call for EMS may be made under false pretenses (e.g., an assault called in as a fall) initially. Although questioning the patient and bystanders may reveal the possibility of domestic assault, it is not the EMS practitioner's responsibility to confront the assailant. This is a very dangerous action. Unfortunately, EMS practitioners encounter domestic violence and the victims involved. You may arrive on a scene while the violence is occurring. As you enter any scene, you should listen for yelling, sounds of a struggle, the breaking of items, and other out-of-the-ordinary noises. If you suspect the possibility of domestic violence during your scene size-up, do not knock on the door or do anything that could alert the perpetrator to your presence. Use the three Rs: retreat to a safe location, radio for assistance from law enforcement, and reassess the situation. If you entered what you consider to be a safe scene, be aware of the bystanders in the room and surrounding rooms because the perpetrator may still be present or might return to the scene while you are still there. Ask all bystanders to vacate the room and ensure that they do not block your egress path. Keep track of where your partner is at all times. Remove the patient to the ambulance as soon as possible.
- **Desperate.** Desperate patients are not always patients with a long history of behavioral or psychiatric issues; instead, they may be everyday people who are lonely, who feel helpless, and who are unable to endure the pain that they are feeling right now. Desperation may drive some people to perform acts they would not normally do, and this includes violent acts against EMS practitioners. Patients who are experiencing desperation will present with behavioral warning signs such as agitation, yelling, or even making verbal threats. As noted earlier, use your communication skills to de-escalate the tension, follow your local protocols, and contact law enforcement if you feel that your safety or the safety of others is at risk.
- **Bonus D: "Don't know."** There have been several cases in which EMS or fire personnel have

been shot and killed while responding to relatively mundane "welfare checks" or medical alarms. If dispatch is not able to get information from a caller or the caller is getting agitated or angry at them, do not hesitate to request the presence of law enforcement.

In the Field

Stating or documenting that a patient is "drunk" may be considered slander or libel, and it is not a diagnosis, but more of an assumption. A person who is known to have ingested alcohol may in fact be "drunk," but remember that all medical possibilities of the cause of an intoxicated patient's altered mental status must be ruled out during the patient assessment process. Providing a blood alcohol level, if available, is more accurate.

Delirium With Agitated Behavior

The term "excited delirium" is not universally recognized by the medical community. Therefore, delirium with agitated or combative behavior is the term used to describe a condition in which a patient has confused thinking and a reduced awareness of their environment. **Delirium with agitated behavior** is a true medical emergency that has the potential to be fatal if inappropriately managed. Statistically, males are at greater risk for this condition. Other risk factors include the use of stimulant drugs, such as bath salts, cocaine, methamphetamine (meth), PCP, or lysergic acid diethylamide (LSD), and a history of schizophrenia or bipolar disorder. The onset is acute, and EMS practitioner safety is of greatest concern. These patients have an increased sympathetic response (fight-or-flight response) and may become agitated, violent, combative, or paranoid. Patients may present with psychotic symptoms (including hallucinations), have an increase in strength, and become insensitive to pain or self-inflicted injuries.

Suspect delirium if the patient is sweating profusely and hallucinating or presenting with psychotic symptoms (**FIGURE 6-8**). The patient with delirium may disrobe or have already disrobed prior to your arrival due to extreme body temperature. Clinical conditions associated with patient agitation include hyperthermia, tachycardia, tachypnea, hypertension, rhabdomyolysis, and cardiac arrest.

The response to a patient who has delirium with agitated behavior should be based on agency protocols.

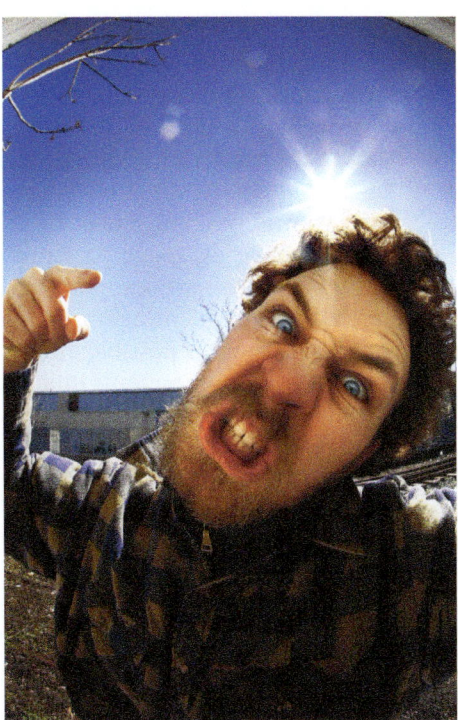

FIGURE 6-8 A patient with suspected delirium with agitated behavior can be very dangerous.
© 9387388673/Shutterstock.

In the Field

Patients who have delirium with agitated or combative behavior may not respond to verbal de-escalation tactics. They often have varying mood swings; do not assume that the patient with suspected delirium who is momentarily calm and cooperative will maintain that demeanor.

Ideally, the EMS agency will have a patient-centered clinical protocol for management of agitated patients that has been approved by the agency medical director. If EMS practitioners arrive on scene of a suspected patient with excited delirium before the arrival of law enforcement and feel they are in danger of harm, they should retreat to a safe area and await law enforcement's arrival. Policies should be in place regarding the role that each agency will take and what is expected of each agency to work cooperatively when managing a patient who is agitated or combative and in need of medical care.

Excited delirium may mimic medical conditions that cause altered mental status such as hypoglycemia, psychiatric crisis, and thyroid disorders. Use the AEIOU-TIPS mnemonic to rule out other causes.

EMS practitioners should follow their local policies regarding the management of patients with excited delirium. If physical restraint is part of local policies, remember that the restraint process is dangerous; the extreme physical exertion may cause cardiac arrest and sudden death in the patient. Never allow your patients to be placed in the prone position, never tie their extremities together, or have excessive pressure put on their backs. These procedures are known to cause *positional asphyxia*, leading to patient death. Be prepared to sedate the patient as soon as possible after physical restraint and cool hyperthermic patients quickly. Monitor the patient's vital signs closely and continuously.

Patient Restraint

EMS practitioners should familiarize themselves with their agency's protocol on the restraint of a patient. Healthcare personnel should maintain awareness of medical-legal risks that could arise from the use of restraints (e.g., consent, duty to protect, battery/false imprisonment, and duty to warn are some examples). EMS agencies should have policies and procedures in effect that have taken into account all local, regional, state, and federal guidelines. The policies and procedures should be reviewed by the agency's legal department. Employee training on patient restraint should be consistent and ongoing.

Agitated, combative, and violent patients may require some sort of restraint during prehospital care to protect themselves, the public, and the responding EMS practitioners, as well as to facilitate assessment or to allow for the treatment of a life-threatening illness or injury. However, remember that EMS practitioners do not attempt to restrain a person who is purposefully violent; that person is not a patient. If they are an attacker and you are trying to "control" them or take "custody" rather than escaping the violent encounter, you are putting yourself at increased liability. If restraints are required, every precaution should be taken to ensure the safety of both the emergency responders and the patient. The restraints used should provide some form of dignity to the patient, and you should be able to quickly remove them if patient care dictates it. Patients should *never* be sandwiched between two devices as a restraint and should *never* be positioned prone. Both of these methods prevent rapid access to the patient's airway and may cause respiratory compromise or respiratory arrest. Handcuffs are not medical restraints, and their use is discouraged. Instead, the use of soft restraints is encouraged. If the patient is in custody of police and is handcuffed, a law enforcement officer with a key should ride with the patient.

Patients might continue to struggle even after being restrained. Struggling while restrained may create additional problems for the patient and EMS practitioners. The patient may develop hyperkalemia, rhabdomyolysis, and respiratory or cardiac arrest. Carefully monitor and reassess your patient and follow your local policies.

Law enforcement should be requested to the scene, and medical control should be contacted before attempting patient restraint. Ensure that enough trained personnel are available to perform the restraint process safely; a minimum of five people is required—one for each limb and one for the head—but six are preferred because someone is needed for the application of the restraint device. If these recommendations cannot be met, it is best to withdraw from the immediate scene and await law enforcement and additional personnel. Be sure to document the incident with as much detail as possible. Begin with your assessment findings, a description of the patient's behavior, any attempts that were made to de-escalate the situation or gain the patient's cooperation, and the restraint method chosen. Be sure to document a continued assessment and monitoring of the patient.

Stay in the Field

Assisting in restraining a patient can be dangerous for EMS practitioners. It is vital that you maintain your training, follow local policies, and ensure that the proper number of emergency responders is on hand before restraint is attempted.

Pharmacologic Management/ Sedation

Pharmacologic sedation is the use of medications to manage an agitated, combative, or violent patient to prevent self-harm. The following medications are commonly used: (1) dissociative anesthetic (e.g., ketamine), (2) benzodiazepine (e.g., midazolam), (3) butyrophenone (e.g., droperidol), or (4) a combination of these. Know your available sedative agent's pharmacologic properties (indications, contraindications, and side effects). These agents are generally indicated if performing physical restraint as a medical intervention. Respiratory depression can be a serious side effect that must be closely monitored for and can be remedied with airway adjuncts, oxygen, and in the worst-case scenario, ventilations. Pharmacologic management should not be used at the request of law enforcement, as it is a medical decision. If in doubt, consult with medical control.

Restraint Documentation

Detailed documentation is essential for all patient care reports. If it becomes necessary to physically restrain or pharmacologically manage a patient, your documentation on the PCR should include the following:

- Assessment findings
- Description of the patient's behavior
- Clinical indication for the restraint
- Attempts made to de-escalate the situation or gain the patient's cooperation
- Method of restraint selected
- Continued assessment frequency and any exam findings
- Additional care provided throughout transport
- Scores on any patient assessment scales used (e.g., Richmond Agitation-Sedation Scale)

Restraint Pitfalls

Some of the common pitfalls of patient restraint by EMS practitioners include the following:

- Lack of restraint training for the individual and for the organization (e.g., cooperative training).
- Failure to recognize patients at risk of excited delirium or positional asphyxia.
- Failure to provide the appropriate care and reassessment of restrained patients.
- Failure to report injuries inflicted on EMS practitioners.

Agency Actions and Resources

Your agency needs to act now to prevent injuries or death occurring to EMS practitioners. This requires a total culture of safety, as emphasized throughout this text and the EMS Safety course. Training and policies were identified as the top two items found to be deficient in a 2019 NAEMT violence survey. Reporting assaults could highlight the problem and lead to EMS provider assistance, in particular the mental health aspect that violence has on EMS practitioners. It should not take the death of an EMS provider to institute a forever change!

The 2019 study also reported that approximately 57% to 93% of EMS practitioner have been physically or verbally assaulted at least once in their career. The SAVER (Stress and Violence in EMS Responders) checklist includes 174 items organized into six phases that support what organizations can do to mitigate violence in EMS. Specific actions for organizational leadership to introduce could be completed through policy, environmental, and training modifications. The six phases are as follows:

- **Pre-event.** Policies, procedures, and training that can be effective in mitigating harm
- **Traveling to the scene.** Preplanning en route, dispatch protocols, law enforcement assist
- **Scene arrival.** Staging, body armor, dispatch protocols/communication with law enforcement
- **Patient care.** Care policies, restraint policies, and tools
- **Readiness to return to service.** Physical and emotional support for the EMS crew immediately after the call
- **Post event.** Incident reporting, ongoing mental health support for court appearances

Summary

Every scene has the potential for violence. Scene size-up is always dynamic and ever changing, so maintaining situational awareness on all scenes is critical. Use nonverbal and verbal communication techniques for de-escalation. Determine whether restraints, physical and/or pharmacologic, are required to ensure patient and responder safety. EMS agencies must design and employ systems that minimize risks to EMS practitioners and patients. Finally, above all, your safety is most important!

CHAPTER WRAP-UP

- Every scene has the potential for violence.
- Situational awareness on all scenes is critical.
- Use nonverbal and verbal communication techniques for de-escalation.
- If restraints—physical and/or pharmacologic—are required, ensure patient and responder safety.
- Above all, your safety is most important!

SUMMARY

- Every emergency scene has the potential to create an unsafe environment for EMS practitioners. Remember that scene size-up is a dynamic, evolving practice, and never take anything for granted.

- Any type of response could be a potential crime scene. All crime scenes have the potential to be dangerous, but active crime scenes have an increased risk. Whenever possible, move your patient to the ambulance and, if necessary, drive around the corner to a safe location to continue patient care.

- Patients from secure facilities with behavioral or mental health concerns are sometimes outwardly violent to EMS practitioners, and practitioners should take appropriate precautions per local policies and procedures to prevent personal injury.

- While within a secure facility, follow the directions of staff, and do not be afraid to ask questions.

- EMS practitioners should have a basic understanding of weapons and how to safeguard them if found during a call or when treating a law enforcement officer.

- To effectively and safely communicate with patients, family members, and bystanders, EMS practitioners must develop a thorough understanding of verbal and physical or nonverbal communication. How you say something, what you say, and how you look when say it can affect how the patient responds to you and how much information you are able to elicit.

- Poor communication may compromise patient care and put EMS practitioners at risk.

- Communication works two ways. EMS practitioners must learn not only to communicate effectively but also to "read" the patient and bystanders around them.

- Likely scenes for violence include those involving the six Ds: drunk, drugged, diabetic, deranged, domestic, and desperate.

- Patients who have delirium with agitated behavior are experiencing a fight-or-flight response and may become agitated, violent, combative, or paranoid.

- The response to a patient who has delirium with agitated behavior should be a tiered, multiagency one. EMS agencies should have a documented response policy.

- Agitated, combative, and violent patients may require some sort of restraint during the prehospital care phase. If restraints are required, every precaution should be taken to ensure the safety of both the emergency responders and the patient. Be sure to document a continued assessment and monitoring of the patient.

GLOSSARY

assessment "L" formation A formation that permits one EMS practitioner to address the patient from the front and another EMS practitioner to remain at the patient's side, performing patient care. If the patient attacks, this formation provides the second EMS practitioner enough time to escape and call for help.

concealment An object that hides a person from view but does not protect him or her from projectiles or a potential attacker.

cover A barrier that both hides and protects—for example, a brick wall, large rocks, or a vehicle engine block.

defensive stance A position that creates a nonthreatening, nonaggressive appearance. The EMS practitioner stands with hands up and palms forward in an open position, keeping the elbows in and angling the body 45 degrees to the patient.

delirium with agitated behavior A condition in which patients have an increased sympathetic response and may become agitated, violent, combative, or paranoid.

pharmacologic sedation The use of medications to manage an agitated, combative, or violent patient to prevent self-harm.

surveying stance The body posture to take when defusing a stressful patient encounter. The body is slightly at an angle, with hands above the waist and out of the pockets, arms neutral, and knees slightly bent with the weight on the balls of the feet.

REFERENCES

American College of Surgeons. The Hartford Consensus. Accessed November 28, 2020. https://www.facs.org/about-acs/hartford-consensus

Center for Firefighter Injury Research and Safety Trends. Stress and Violence in Fire-Based EMS Responders (SAVER) Systems-Level Checklist. Accessed April 9, 2021. https://drexel.edu/~/media/Files/dornsife/FIRST/Projects/SAVER%20Items/CKlist%20manuscript_FDSOA_FINAL%20for%20website.ashx?la=en

DT4EMS. How can removing the words "combative patient" reduce workplace violence in medicine? Accessed December 9, 2021. http://dt4ems.com/how-often-do-you-really-deal-with-a-combative-patient/

EMS Behavioral Restraint 2019 - Physical Restraint Application Procedure. YouTube. Revised November 2019. Accessed April 10, 2021. https://www.youtube.com/watch?v=3Dk5EQ02gvU

Goodwin J, NAEMT EMS Workforce Committee. Violence against EMS practitioners. Accessed April 9, 2021. https://www.naemt.org/docs/default-source/2017-publication-docs/naemt-violence-report-web-10-02-2019.pdf?Status=Temp&sfvrsn=b700d792_2

Kupas DF, Wydro GC, Tan DK, Kamin R, Harrell AJ, Wang A. Clinical care and restraint of agitated or combative patients by emergency medical services practitioners. *Prehosp Emerg Care.* 2021 Apr 20;25(5):721-723. doi:10.1080/10903127.2021.1917736

National Association of Emergency Medical Technicians. *Experiences with Emergency Medical Services Survey.* Clinton, MS: NAEMT; 2005.

National Institute for Occupational Safety and Health. Career Fire Fighter Killed and Volunteer Fire Fighter Seriously Wounded When Shot during a Civilian Welfare Check—Maryland. Published October 10, 2018. Accessed April 9, 2021. https://www.cdc.gov/niosh/fire/pdfs/face201606.pdf

Natoli S. 6 Ways to Improve Your Non-verbal Communication Skills. Mental Health First Aid. Published June 18, 2018. https://www.mentalhealthfirstaid.org/external/2018/06/6-ways-to-improve-your-non-verbal-communication-skills/

Reichard AA, Marsh SM, Tonozzi TR, Konda S, Gormley MA. Occupational injuries and exposures among emergency medical services workers. *Prehosp Emerg Care.* 2017;21(4):420-431. doi:10.1080/10903127.2016.1274350

Taylor JA, Murray RM, Davis AL, et al. Creation of a systems-level checklist to address stress and violence in fire-based emergency medical services responders. *Occup Health Sci.* 2019;3(3):265-295. doi:10.1007/s41542-019-00047-z

Thomas J, Moore G. Medical-legal issues in the agitated patient: cases and caveats. *West J Emerg Med.* 2013;14(5):559-565. doi:10.5811/westjem.2013.4.16132

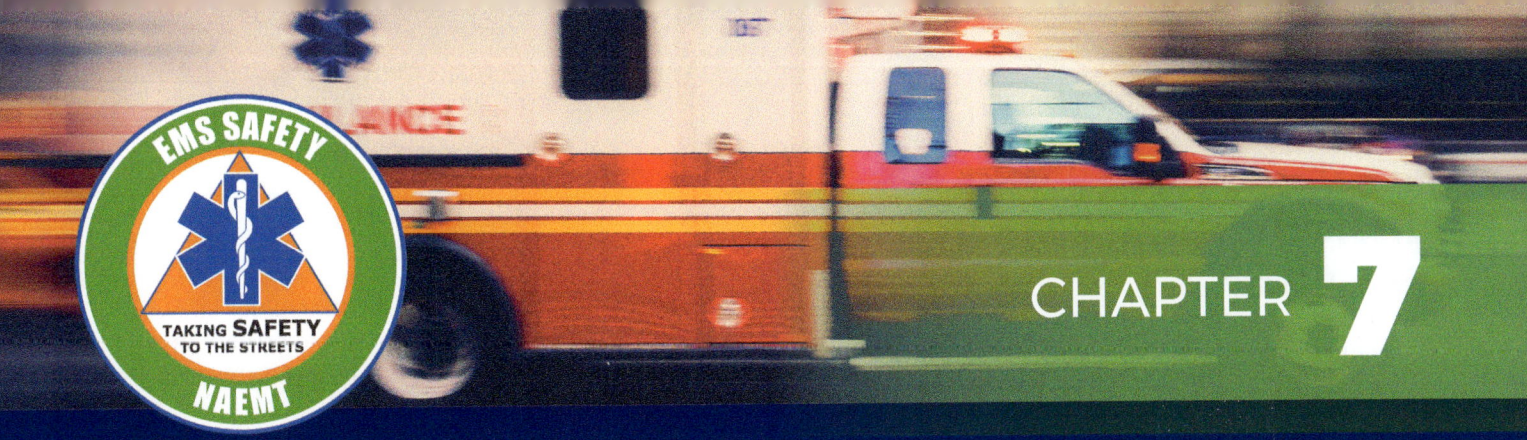

CHAPTER 7

Injury and Infection Prevention

LESON OBJECTIVES

- Discuss common causes of injuries to EMS practitioners.
- Recognize EMS practitioner risk for back injuries.
- Demonstrate a safe lifting and moving plan.
- Discuss the importance of standard precautions and source control as it relates to infection prevention.

- Identify the different levels of isolation precautions and the corresponding personal protective equipment.
- Describe ways to maintain EMS practitioner safety while providing care to patients with new or drug-resistant organisms.

Scenario

You and your partner get a late call, about 11:45 p.m. on a night when you are scheduled until midnight and hoping to get out on time. There is no sign of the oncoming crew, so you head out to an address you have been to many times before. The patient is an elderly male with COPD who is always grouchy and argumentative. He lives with his daughter who is concerned because her dad is short of breath again tonight. It has been a very hot evening and their small air conditioner is not adequately cooling the apartment. As on most previous calls, Mr. Stone does not want to go to the hospital, although he is obviously short of breath. After taking his vitals and updating his history, you are able to convince him to go in the ambulance. It takes more convincing to talk him into getting on the stair chair, rather than walking down a flight of stairs. Meanwhile, the relief crew will not be meeting you at the scene, because they have already been dispatched to another call. Mr. Stone refused a metered-dose inhaler (MDI) treatment, even though all the while he is coughing on you. Mr. Stone then argues about the chest straps for the stair chair ride. You decide to let him have his arms free since it is just one flight of steps, and all the arguing with him is getting under your skin.

Halfway down the stairway, using one of those older-style stair chairs without the treads, he gets nervous and reaches out to grab the railing. Luckily, your partner notices right away and yells at him not to touch the railing: "Put your hands on your chest!" Mr. Stone follows the command and seems to calm down for the rest of the call and during the ride to the hospital.

1. What are some of the stressors that led to a poor decision in this case?
2. Why should the patient's hands be strapped in for the ride?
3. What is the advantage of the tread-style stair chairs over the older style?

Introduction: EMS Injuries

The field of EMS puts its practitioners in potentially dangerous situations that can cause occupational injury and/or increased risk of illness. Both the agency leadership and the practitioners must take an ongoing responsibility to understand the hazards and reduce the risks as much as possible. According to the U.S. Bureau of Labor Statistics, based on 2019 data, the rate of injuries and illness in nongovernmental emergency medical services (EMS) is 7.9 injuries/illnesses per 100 full-time employees, as compared to the U.S. average of 2.8 per 100 full-time employees. The rate of cases involving days missed at work, job restriction, or transfer is 4.5 per 100 full-time employees compared to the U.S. average of 1.5 per 100 full-time employees. In fact, the rate of musculoskeletal disorders for EMS practitioners is six times higher than the national average. These injury rates are all significantly higher than general industry in the United States

Stay in the Field

A 2017 study looked at the demographics of injured EMS workers who sought treatment in an emergency department (ED). The study revealed the following:

- Two-thirds were male.
- 52% had less than 10 years' experience.
- 42% were 18 to 29 years old.
- 15% were permanently impaired by the injury.
- Workers age 40 years or older had the highest injury rates.
- Sprains and strains accounted for 40% of injuries. Of these injuries, 90% occurred while lifting, carrying, or transferring a patient and/or equipment.

Data from Reichard AA, Marsh SM, Tonozzi TR, Konda S, Gormley MA. Occupational injuries and exposures among emergency medical services workers. *Prehosp Emerg Care*. 2017;21(4):420-431. doi: 10.1080/10903127.2016.1274350

Injury Causes

The causes of injuries to EMS practitioners fall primarily into five categories: body motion; exposure to harmful substances; slips, trips and falls; motor vehicle incidents; and violence and assaults. Specifically, the most common work injuries in EMS were due to body motion, which includes excessive physical effort, awkward posture, or repetitive motion. When reviewed, most EMS practitioners were injured during transfer, carrying, or lifting of a patient. In the exposure to harmful substance category, most exposures were incidents involving blood or respiratory secretions, with approximately one-fifth of the exposure incidents resulting from needlestick injuries.

About 40% of injuries in the slips, trips, and fall category were incurred when going up or down steps or curbs. Other injuries in this category were caused by getting into or out of the ambulance. Motor vehicle incidents included two-thirds of the injuries caused from a collision with other vehicles. Reports of violence and assaults were common; however, this category is thought to be highly underreported by EMS personnel. In most cases the assailant was the patient being cared for, with almost half appearing to be intoxicated.

According to a 2007 article in the *American Journal of Industrial Medicine*, about 10% of the EMS workforce is on leave at any given time because of illness or injury. Unfortunately, this number is currently cited as accurate.

There is an apparent epidemic of back injuries in EMS. Consider the following:

- Back injury is the top reason for seeing a doctor.
- Back injury is the most common cause of disability.
- Half of all EMS practitioners are affected by some degree of back injury.
- Back injury is the top reason for leaving EMS.
- Back injury is often the result of cumulative wear and tear.

The occurrence of back injury has been related to high call volume, which in this context was defined as 40 or more calls per week. EMS workers in communities with a population of 25,000 or more were three times more likely to report an injury than those in a rural environment.

Critical Risk Factors

A number of contributors to back injuries have been identified. Uncoordinated lifts are a risk factor and can occur when one practitioner is lowering the stretcher while the other practitioner is trying to raise the stretcher. Anthropometric disparities may exist in lifting pairs (e.g., differences in height, strength, arm length, etc.) that can increase the risk of injury to one or both practitioners. Many safety-sensitive functions (e.g., balance, fine motor coordination, judgment) that are critical risk factors can contribute to injury. An injured team member may be concealing their weakness or disability, and this can present a higher risk of injury to themselves and the other members of the team. Untrained lifters may inadvertently cause injuries to other team members because of their knowledge deficit. It is imperative that organization leadership ensure that all team members are trained properly in lifting safety techniques. Poor communication is another risk factor that can contribute to injury. Does "lift on three" mean that the team lifts after the one-two-three count or when three is being stated? Perhaps a better solution would be a command of "Ready, set, lift, and we will actually start lifting when I say lift." Finally, poor physical conditioning of one of the EMS practitioners can contribute to the risk of injury.

Stay in the Field

A quality fitness program can make you stronger. Many EMS practitioners with weak abdominal, pelvic, hip, and gluteal muscles lack the endurance to do their job throughout the day, so they place an extra load on the muscles of the spine and back. Keeping your core strong is important in protecting your back.

You should exercise to increase your endurance, but strength alone will not keep you injury-free. You need to have the strength to do your job, but you also need the flexibility. To keep your muscles active, functioning, and ready to lift, it is vital to stretch at the beginning of your shift and several times throughout. Flexibility and mobility increase with stretching and elongating the muscles that shorten when they are not being used. Feet, ankles, hamstrings, hip flexors, and pectoral and gluteal muscles are your workhorses. No one would expect to run a marathon without proper stretching and maintenance, yet EMS practitioners expect their bodies to be in peak performance on the job without taking care of them. Quite often EMS practitioners take better care of their vehicles than their bodies, and expect their bodies to last throughout their careers.

Direct and Indirect Costs of Back Injuries

Work-related injury is expensive and includes both direct and indirect costs that are not covered entirely by your workers' compensation insurance benefits.

Direct costs are those commonly associated with out-of-pocket payments. They include payments to physicians, rehabilitation professionals, insurance carriers, and attorneys. Other direct costs are compensatory salaries for lost work and employee replacement costs (often at the overtime rate). The financial impact to an EMS practitioner can be devastating.

In terms of actual dollars, it is estimated that a simple lumbar sprain will have an average direct cost of $18,365. A more complicated back injury can have direct costs of $100,000 per year. Subsequent back injuries can cost two to four times the cost of the first injury.

One way to look at direct costs is to think of them as what it takes to make the physical pain and disability go away. It seems that it would be smarter to avoid the pain and disability, skip the suffering, and save the money through utilizing preventive techniques that minimize lifting, such as lift assist teams and patient-handling equipment and devices. Never be too proud to ask for a lift assist, and always avoid complacency when planning a lift.

Indirect costs may be 15 to 40 times greater than direct costs. Indirect costs are those expenses that society incurs when you have a debilitating injury that does not allow you to be you. Your inability to function at home costs money and creates psychological pain for your family. How does your injury alter the way your significant other and children live? What adaptations do they have to make? How many EMS practitioners work multiple jobs or take as much overtime as possible just to make ends meet? What happens if your household must manage solely on disability income, which is usually around two-thirds of base pay?

In addition, there are the indirect costs that can change how you feel about yourself and your lifestyle. Most EMS practitioners describe themselves as very independent people. Examples of indirect costs include the following:

- A loss of independence due to injury can be very troubling to the injured worker.
- Inability to function normally at home and work could result in significant psychological, interpersonal, and financial stress.
- One study indicated that more than one-third of injured EMS practitioners who sought treatment in an ED received pain medication or a muscle relaxant for treatment.
- The combination of loss of self-esteem, pain from an injury, strained interpersonal relationships, and financial stress could present a risk for long-term conditions such as medication dependence or depression.

Remember, it is better to ask for a lift assist with a heavy patient rather than be too proud to ask and risk your own life or a career-changing back injury!

A Complicated Psychomotor Skill

A National Institute of Occupational Safety and Health (NIOSH) study recommends limiting repeatedly lifting weights of more than 51 lb from the ground level. That 51-lb weight places 764 lb of compressive load on the spine. NIOSH developed a lifting equation that calculates the recommended weight limit that workers could lift over an 8-hour shift without increasing their risk of musculoskeletal injury. The equation used 51 lb as the maximum weight that workers should be repeatedly lifting from floor level. Ask most EMS practitioners and they will tell you that 51 lb is not even comparable to the weight they regularly lift. EMS practitioners must find ways to reduce the load. EMS practitioners must learn to lift smarter when lifting off the ground. Use an "all hands lift" culture when lifting from the ground level. Use your lifting device, and do not be complacent (e.g., it was only about five or six steps to carry the patient and stretcher rather than taking the time to use the stair chair.)

Patient handling is a complicated psychomotor skill that requires training and practice. Body mechanics classes and training in lifting techniques can help reduce injuries, but retraining is needed on a regular basis. To prevent injury, you should do the following:

- Practice behavior modification. Evaluate and monitor your patient-handling techniques.
- Maintain a healthy body, flexibility, and mobility.
- Carefully review and purchase task-specific equipment and ensure that personnel have the proper training in that equipment.
- Seek out the best practices in injury reduction and prevention.

Although EMS practitioners cannot eliminate lifting, you can identify situations that pose a higher risk and use extra personnel and equipment to minimize that risk.

Stay in the Field

Myth: Back injuries usually happen when lifting obese patients.

Facts: Most injuries occur during a routine call.

With heavier patients, EMS practitioners actually place a more significant emphasis on lifting techniques. Oftentimes, EMS practitioners do not think through a lift if it is routine. The 90-lb patient whom you think will not be a problem

lifting is quite often the one who injures the EMS practitioner. EMS practitioners typically do not think about or prepare for a smaller lift as they would for a heavier patient. EMS practitioners use improper technique and often move too quickly. Use of equipment such as a slide sheet or patient mover should be a common practice even with routine transfers. Ironically, 64% of the injuries involving treatment of EMS practitioners in an ED occurred on calls where no lifting assistance was present, according to a 2017 study that looked at the demographics of injured EMS workers.

Patient Handling and Crew Resource Management

The principals of crew resource management (CRM) can be applied to patient handling. CRM is discussed in greater detail in Chapter 2, *Crew Resource Management.*

Situational awareness is not just about scene safety. EMS practitioners must evaluate and constantly be alert to changing circumstances when moving a patient. For example, both moving a patient to the ambulance through rough terrain or having a stretcher wheel get caught in a storm grate can lead to tipping over.

In the Field

Injury and illness data for EMS workers reveals that most of the injuries (sprains and strains) involved bodily reactions and exertion. Approximately one-half of the overexertion events occurred during lifting. Surprisingly, a study in the *Journal of Occupational Medicine* showed that although classes in body mechanics and training in lifting techniques improved skills in the short term, alone they do not reduce injuries. Follow-up studies show that emphasizing the use of task-specific patient-handling equipment, such as power cots, antifriction devices, and bariatric devices, were mandatory, along with body mechanics training, for achieving a successful injury prevention program. The proper use of lifting and moving equipment requires training and retraining for EMS practitioners.

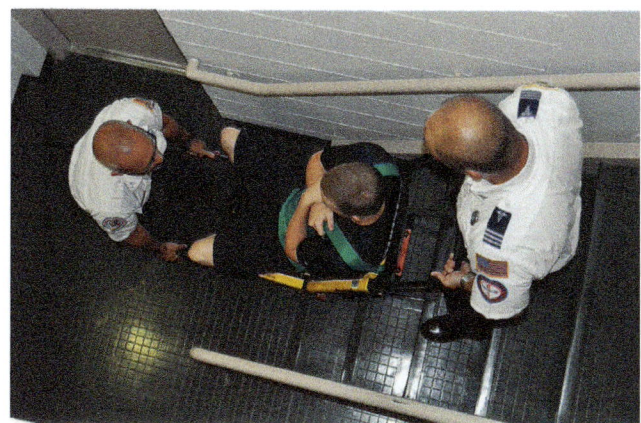

FIGURE 7-1 Properly using equipment such as a stair chair can help protect your back.
Courtesy of Sunstar Paramedics.

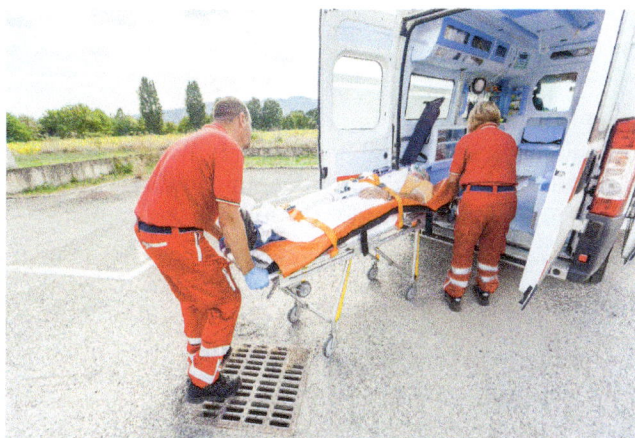

FIGURE 7-2 Anticipate everything that could happen during the move and use critical thinking skills when planning a lift.
© William Perugini/Shutterstock.

Although EMS practitioners cannot completely eliminate lifting, they can identify lifting situations with higher risks and use task-specific patient-handling equipment with proper body mechanics to minimize the cumulative and acute effects of lifting—for example, using a stair chair rather than carrying a patient down stairs (**FIGURE 7-1**).

In addition, EMS practitioners cannot maintain the misconception that injuries occur only with strenuous lifting. Injuries can and do occur during "routine" lifting, such as moving a 90-lb nursing home patient from a bed to a stretcher. EMS practitioners must use situational awareness and treat each lifting event as a potential source of injury.

Use critical thinking skills when planning a lift. An example would be to determine if it would be better to lift the patient over the terrain instead of trying to push the stretcher through it. Anticipate everything that could happen during the move (**FIGURE 7-2**). Ensure

that the patient is informed continuously of what is going to happen throughout the move to minimize panic and unpredictable actions. Remember, if you see something, say something. Most EMS practitioners who had a stretcher tip over saw an unsafe behavior prior to the event and did nothing to avoid it.

Safe Patient Movement Behavior

Safe patient movement combines evidence-based practices, training, body maintenance, and common sense. It has been shown that formal patient lifting classes in body mechanics and training in safe lifting techniques do not reduce caregiver injuries by themselves. Training is important, but it must be combined with evidence-based practices to be effective. Evidence-based practices include the following:

- Minimizing manual patient handling
- Utilizing lift assist and lift teams
- Employing patient and environment assessment strategies
- Utilizing patient-handling equipment and devices
- Training and retraining on lifting and equipment use
- Engaging in behavior modification
- Maintaining a healthy body, including flexibility and mobility

Behavioral Controls

Safe patient movement requires the selection of **safe patient movement behaviors**. These behaviors involve movement actions selected by the EMS practitioner that minimize the risk of injury to patients, practitioners, and bystanders during patient movement events. They include the proper evaluation of the patient and environment, acquisition of adequate resources (properly trained personnel and appropriate equipment), the use of proper body mechanics, and ongoing communication among team members and the patient. This is achieved in part through the implementation of behavioral controls.

Behavioral controls are techniques to promote injury prevention and reduction, and they include providing the following:

- Training on the necessary cognitive and psychomotor skills for lifting
- Management oversight, enforcement, and a culture of safety that makes employees want to use the available resources
- Primary training in appropriate body mechanics and effective lifting techniques

Behavioral controls require management oversight (standard operating procedures [SOPs]), enforcement (compliance with safety standards), and a culture of safety that makes employees want to use the available resources. In an organization with a culture of safety, everyone in the organization feels empowered to stop unsafe actions and to offer opinions on different ways to accomplish a task. Patient and environmental assessments are examples of behavioral controls. Education and training are not effective if the desired behaviors do not exist. EMS practitioners should take pride and ownership in how a patient is handled and treated.

Safe patient movement behaviors can only be performed by EMS practitioners who know what to do, are physically capable of doing it, and, most important, want to do it safely.

Stay in the Field

When moving a patient, do not forget to use proper body mechanics each and every time. Proper body mechanics should be a habit so that when something goes wrong, your muscle memory kicks in and maintains the best form and technique. Proper body mechanics include the following:

- Keeping your head up and shoulders back
- Keeping your eyes on your partner's face
- Maintaining abdominal bracing (stiffening your core to apply pressure on your spine)
- Keeping your feet rooted to the floor, slightly wider than shoulder width, and toes pointed slightly outward
- Keeping your hips hinged and not pushed forward, so you can do a proper squat
- Keeping your palms faceup
- Keeping the load close to your body

Your injury prevention and reduction should include regularly scheduled refresher training to review all lifting equipment used by your agency and providing and encouraging fitness training. Some agencies have been able to either negotiate gym membership discounts with local gyms or have purchased fitness equipment for their agency personnel's use. There also needs to be education and training in the proper use and selection of **engineering controls**, that is, the tools designed to make a task safer or easier or changes made to the work environment through the use of equipment to avoid work-related injury. EMS-specific engineering controls include powered stretchers/load systems, stair chairs, sharps protection, and so forth. Preshift factors are also important to injury prevention and reduction. Having a proper amount of rest prior to a shift is imperative, because fatigue can impair motor coordination, balance, and judgment. Nutrition also plays a pivotal role in ensuring practitioners have the energy and stamina to perform strenuous activities such as patient handling while on long-duration shifts. Finally, providing clinical tools such as assessment protocols and algorithms that can give EMS practitioners a heads-up to help plan the move.

Evaluation of the Patient and Environment

Evaluate the Patient

What do EMS practitioners need to know about the patient before they can move him or her safely (**FIGURE 7-3**)? In addition to your condition-specific clinical assessment, consider the following:

- Age (spectrum from infant to elderly)
- Ability of the patient to provide assistance (independent, partial, or dependent)
- Ability to bear weight (full, partial, or none)
- Upper extremity strength (bilateral)
- Ability and *willingness* to cooperate and follow instructions (acute chronic cognitive impairment or language barrier)
- Height and weight (body mass index, bariatric, or **cachectic** [possessing an appearance of wasting away])

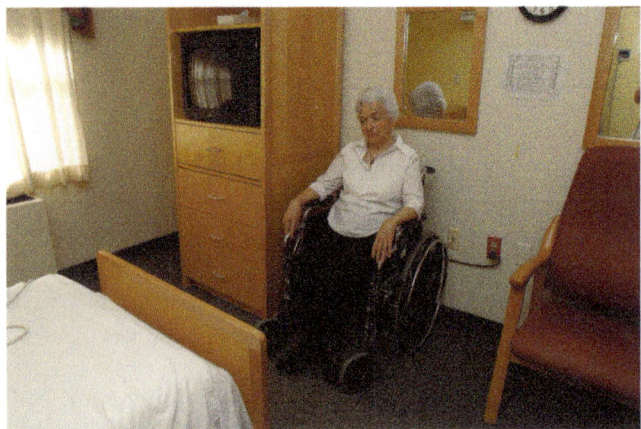

FIGURE 7-3 What do you need to know about this patient before you can move her safely?
© Jones & Bartlett Learning.

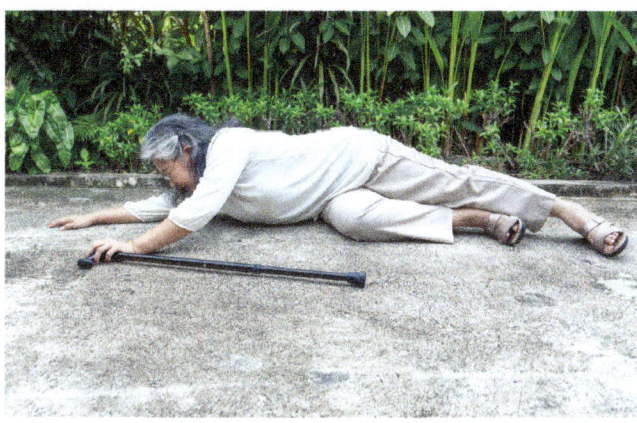

FIGURE 7-4 Evaluate the patient as a part of creating a lifting and moving plan.

© Anatta_Tan/Shutterstock.

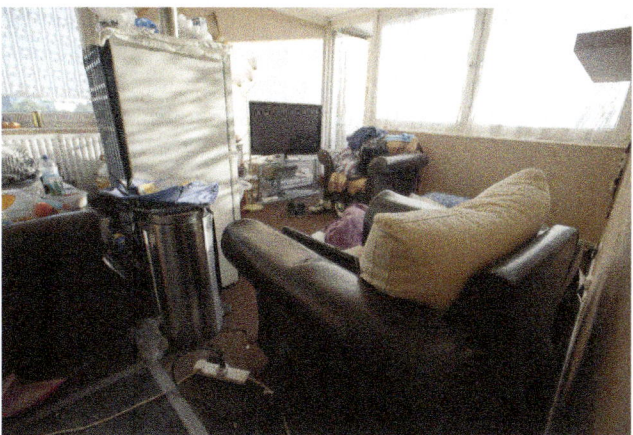

FIGURE 7-5 What are the potential hazards in this environment?

© Ivan Strba/iStock/Getty Images.

Evaluate the patient in **FIGURE 7-4** to determine if there are any special circumstances to consider in a lifting and moving plan, such as the following:

- Conditions likely to affect patient handling, including amputations, spasms, fractures, joint replacement, paralysis, cardiorespiratory compromise, edema, osteoporosis, pain, urinary or fecal stoma, and very fragile skin
- Conditions that increase the risk of a fall, including patient over 65, multiple diagnoses, history of falls over the past 3 months, incontinence, vision impairment, impaired functional mobility, polypharmacy (four or more prescriptions), postural hypotension, and fear of falling
- Special circumstances likely to affect transfer or repositioning tasks, including abdominal wounds, tubes, or other medical equipment that is either attached or implanted
- Specific physician orders that require additional personnel for patient transferring or repositioning, including recent joint replacement or fractures and specific angles of extension of abduction or adduction

After determining the patient's needs, the EMS practitioner must evaluate the environment.

Evaluate the Environment

The EMS practitioner must perform an environmental assessment to determine how the environment will impact safe patient movement (**FIGURE 7-5**). In this evaluation, the EMS practitioner will look for the following:

- Presence of fixed physical obstructions (things that cannot be moved)
- Presence of removable physical obstructions (Is it safe to move this item or is an alternative route more sensible?)

- Terrain that requires lifting and carrying the patient to the transport medium (e.g., stretcher, stair chair)
- Terrain that makes the use of good body mechanics difficult
- Distance the patient must be lifted and/or carried
- Presence of adequate lighting
- Freedom from bystander interference
- Factors that prevent or limit the use of engineering controls (e.g., specialty stretchers, lateral transfer aids)

Have you ever had a patient on a stretcher and, while trying to get the patient to the ambulance, found your path blocked? There are two kinds of obstructions to consider. Fixed physical obstructions are those that cannot be moved. Discovering a fixed obstruction requires us to plan how to get around it. Movable physical obstructions are those that can be removed from your path. Isn't it a good idea to move objects *before* reaching them with a patient on a stretcher?

Is there terrain that requires lifting and carrying the patient to the transport medium? When do you take the stretcher to the patient, or the patient to the stretcher? A stretcher should never be taken up a flight of stairs (or five risers). Think about what is physically easier. If stairs are involved, the added weight of the power cot may make a stair chair a better choice. How far must the patient be lifted or carried? Does the terrain make the use of good body mechanics difficult? A steep or slanted incline, a rough or slick surface, or cramped quarters may make it difficult to get into a proper lifting position. Think of building terrain, not just the outdoors. Is the lighting adequate? Is bystander interference an issue? Are there factors that limit your ability to use equipment? Narrow hallways and small rooms may require us to move the patient to the equipment.

Once EMS practitioners obtain the information from their assessments of the patient and the environment, they are ready to process the information and act on it. EMS practitioners do this by forming a plan.

Patient Preparation

Is there a need for immediate patient removal because of hazards, toxins, fire, hostile bystanders, or other dangers? Is there a clinical indication for "load and go," or do you need to stabilize the patient medically before transport?

Do you need to discuss with the patient, family, or other EMS practitioners the effects of any cognitive, communicative, or physical impairments the patient may be exhibiting? Are there medical equipment issues? Are there any clinical conditions that require special positions? Have you considered language barriers or any special needs?

Conditions that take precedence over patient movement issues include dangerous scenes and critical clinical conditions that require immediate transport. Situational awareness and common sense allow us to recognize physical threats. Protocols and communication with medical control help with the clinical concerns.

The EMS practitioner must establish effective communication with the patient. If dementia or other forms of cognitive impairment make the patient unable to follow directions, precautions such as the use of restraints or the presence of a caretaker may be needed. Do you have a rudimentary understanding of the languages spoken by the patient population? If not, do you have immediate access to an interpreter?

Are there physical impairments that require special positioning? Think about amputation, spasms, fractures, joint replacement, paralysis, cardiorespiratory compromise, edema, osteoporosis, pain, urinary or fecal catheter, and very fragile skin.

Personnel Preparation

The number of personnel needed should be determined *before* the lift is attempted. Perform a test lift to see if the team can safely handle the load of the patient or if backup lifters are needed. Consider the size of the patient and the previously mentioned patient and environmental characteristics.

Decide how many people will be needed in each phase. For example, how many people can initially make physical contact with the patient? What devices will be used to move the patient? If the patient must be transported down stairs, how many people will the staircase accommodate? In addition to the people actually moving the patient, how much backup is needed to provide physical support and guidance?

Lift Assist

In those circumstances that require lifting, a good principle is to share the load by using an adequate number of personnel. The goal of a lift assist is to eliminate critical risk factors that contribute to back injury, including cumulative effects (**FIGURE 7-6**).

Lift assist teams are used to supply adequate people power in the case of a heavy patient or other situations in which help is needed to safely move a patient. A **lift assist team** can be made up of additional responders on the scene, hospital staff, or another ambulance crew called in as backup. The key to a successful lift assist team is practicing good communication. Everyone on the team must understand the lifting and moving plan, his or her role in the plan, and exactly when to begin lifting.

In addition to weight, factors such as a long distance to move the patient from the scene to the ambulance,

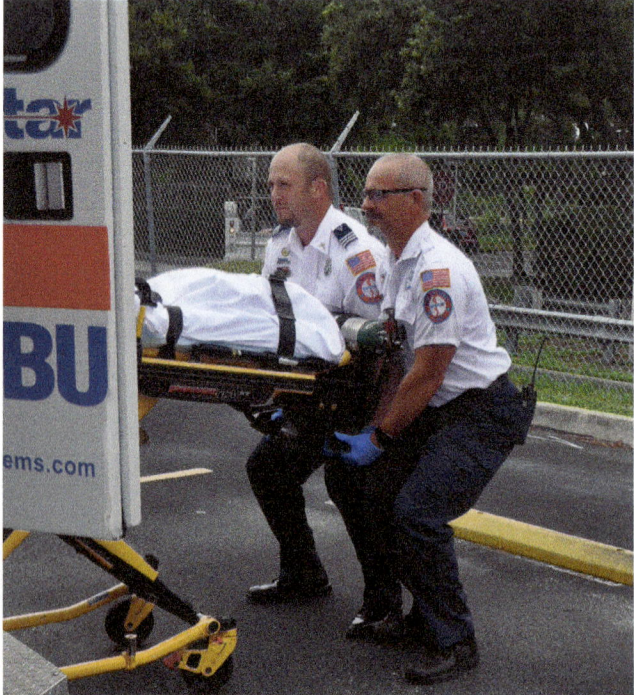

FIGURE 7-6 To prevent injury to the patient or personnel, always share the load.

Courtesy of Sunstar Paramedics.

the presence of ice or snow, and terrain issues such as hills, steps, and other inclines, require assistance. Weight should not be the *only* factor in determining the need for a lift assist.

When in doubt, call for a lift assist.

Stay in the Field

To maximize your safety during a lift, add a verbal "stop" behavior to the prelift count. Instead of counting out "1, 2, 3, Lift," replace it with descriptive commands that incorporate pauses, such as "Ready, Set, Lift." At "Ready," you and your team get into a safe prelift position. At, "Set," you and your team put your heads up, chests up, and prepare to use abdominal bracing during the lift. Then you check your partner to ensure that he or she is in an optimal position, your partner will also check you, and you will all take a breath. Then lift on "Lift." This approach works very well with lift teams, especially with bariatric patients and patients in awkward lifting positions.

Planning and Direction

Once a plan is in place and the team is assembled, the team leader reviews the lifting and moving plan with the team members and the patient. The team leader directs the activities of each team member, including each of the following:

- Lifting
- Use of engineering controls
- Pace of movement while moving to the ambulance
- Loading the patient in the ambulance
- Securing the patient in the ambulance
- Unloading the patient from the ambulance
- Moving the patient to the receiving facility

The risk of uncoordinated lifts by unprotected personnel is straightforward. Disparities occur when there is a size or strength mismatch between partners or among team members that is not taken into consideration before executing the lifting process. Team members who are injured or fatigued and do not share that information make it impossible to safely share the load.

Untrained or nonprofessional lifters should be avoided, but when circumstances mandate their use, they should be given specific instructions, and the team leader should make certain that the instructions are understood.

Poor communication among EMS professionals can be dangerous for the EMS practitioners and the patient. The first time a team lifts a stretcher, a patient

should not be on it. At the beginning of the shift and as part of the inspection process, the ambulance crew should unload and load the stretcher. They should talk about how they will communicate, and describe their preferences and weaknesses; for example, "We will lift on 'Lift' and always make eye contact when communicating." Poor communication results in poor execution. Ambulance crews should engage in regular practice with equipment that is not used frequently.

Stay in the Field

Too often, EMS practitioners rush their lifts and transfers because they hold the erroneous idea that speed will make the movement easier. In many cases, slowing down and breaking up patient lifts into two steps will make the lift safer and reduce the strain on the spine and extremity joints. You should also become familiar with the methods of lateral transfer employed in the hospitals to which you transport. These may include devices such as slider boards, transfer mattresses, or simply draw sheets, which are linen or plastic.

Body Mechanics

The physical condition of the team members, an understanding of the limitations of the physical compatibility of the lifting team, and good communication are mandatory so that all lifters perform the following tasks simultaneously:

- Maintaining balance
- Keeping heads up and eyes looking at the partner's face
- Having all team members in position and acknowledging that they are ready to lift
- Placing all hands on the lifting equipment before the lift
- Using the power grip with the palms up (**FIGURE 7-7**) and hands at least 10 in. apart, palms faceup, and fingers in complete contact with the stretcher bar
- Keeping the feet shoulder-width apart (**FIGURE 7-8**)
- Avoiding twisting
- Bending at the knees to squat
- Maintaining the lumbar curve with the torso upright
- Holding the load close to the body
- Doing a small test lift, lifting the load up and down a few inches to ensure that the team can handle the weight
- Rising slowly

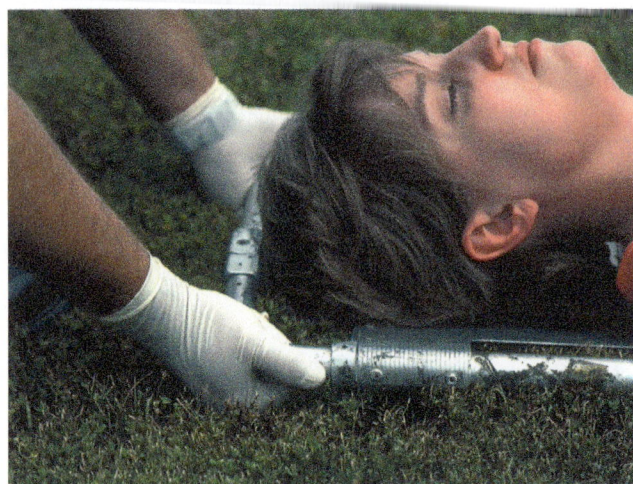

FIGURE 7-7 Use the power grip, with your palms up, when lifting.
© Jones & Bartlett Learning. Courtesy of MIEMSS.

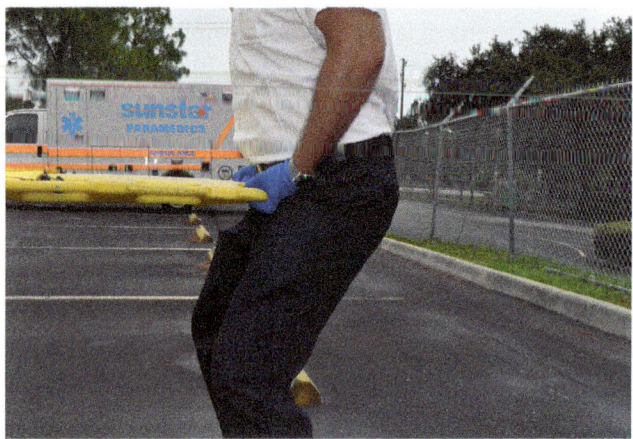

FIGURE 7-8 To protect your back, bend at the knees and keep your feet staggered and shoulder-width apart.
Courtesy of Sunstar Paramedics.

Equipment Maintenance

EMS practitioners have the responsibility to deal with equipment within the limits of their training. This is particularly important with cleaning and maintenance. The increasing complexity of lifting and moving devices requires specialized training to safely maintain and repair this equipment. Keep in mind that the maintenance requirements will vary depending on the equipment. The useful life and length of time it is safe to use a product should be noted at the time of purchase when applicable and tracked by the appropriate management staff in your organization. Maintenance must be performed properly according to the manufacturer's instructions. Service should be performed by a qualified individual. The EMS practitioner must be familiar with the normal functionality of all equipment and immediately report any concerns. Out-of-service equipment should be clearly identified so it is not used until it is repaired.

Preventing Injuries in Vehicles

The risk of occupational injury and death is disproportionately high for EMS practitioners. Many of those casualties are associated with transportation incidents. Ambulances are not built or used in the same manner as standard passenger vehicles. This results in safety concerns for caregivers and patients. While there are inherent risks to occupants in an ambulance, some risks could be reduced by properly restrained occupants and equipment.

Seat Belt Use

Seat belt use is for everyone, not just the patient and the emergency vehicle operator. Of the serious ambulance crashes studied by NIOSH, 84% of EMS personnel in the patient compartment were not restrained. EMS practitioners have plenty of "barriers" to seat belt usage in the patient compartment. Each barrier needs to be discussed and the actions to safely deal with the barrier dealt with. For example, consider the barrier, "I can't reach the IV supplies or medications when I am belted." An example of an action might be, "I can place a soft-sided IV pouch with certain common medications within reach of my seating position in the patient compartment prior to starting transport."

Emergency or not, *every* occupant in the ambulance should always use seat belts while in motion. Most organizational SOPs require restraint use. If your organization's SOP are not clear regarding this issue, your leadership should revisit this important issue. The emergency vehicle operator should take responsibility for ensuring occupant restraint use. Many states mandate driver responsibility. A failure to use provided restraint systems creates risks for all occupants, whether restrained or not. The caregivers and other occupants become projectiles, endangering themselves and others.

Infection Prevention

In the wake of the COVID-19 pandemic there is a renewed commitment to strong infection control practices in EMS. These control practices are accomplished through use of multiple layers of protection, including source control, standard precautions, and transmission-based precautions. Source control is the principle of controlling the spread of potentially infectious material at the source. This can be accomplished by using a surgical mask on the patient, high-efficiency particulate air (HEPA) or bacterial/viral filters on vent circuits, endotracheal tubes, continuous positive airway pressure (CPAP)/bilevel positive airway pressure (BPAP) masks, or a bag-valve mask (BVM). Standard precautions, discussed later in this chapter, include the minimum level of personal protective equipment (PPE) to be worn for each patient contact and work practices to be followed during and after each call (e.g., hand washing, decontamination of medical equipment, sharps safety, proper disposal of contaminated items). Transmission-based precautions include the specific precautions based on the pathogen of concern in addition to standard precautions. This includes contact transmission (both direct and indirect), droplet transmission, and airborne transmission, all of which are discussed later in this chapter.

Source Control

If the patient potentially has an infectious disease that is transmitted via droplet or airborne routes, the patient should wear a mask. If the patient is not wearing a mask on your arrival at the scene and can tolerate one, the mask should be placed on the patient upon initial contact and remain in place throughout transport. Masks, including medical face masks, should not be placed on children younger than 2 years, anyone with trouble breathing, or anyone who is unconscious, incapacitated, or otherwise unable to remove the mask without assistance. Source control can also take the form of a filter on an endotracheal tube, ventilation circuit, CPAP/BiPAP mask, or BVM.

Standard Precautions

Previously called universal precautions or body substance isolation (BSI), the current terminology used is standard precautions. By utilizing the term *standard precautions*, all medical practitioners have the same understanding of the level of precaution that has been initiated. Implementation of standard precautions constitutes the primary strategy for the prevention of healthcare-associated transmission of infectious agents among patients and healthcare personnel.

These precautions are designed to treat all blood and body fluids as potentially infectious. Medical gloves should be worn on all patient contacts, and a gown, mask, goggles/face shield are worn when contact with body fluids is reasonably anticipated. Efforts should be made to minimize exposure to blood or other potentially infectious materials (OPIM). If procedures are to be performed where risk of exposure to blood or OPIM is increased, then the following PPE should be utilized as appropriate: gown, mask, and goggles/face shield.

Transmission-Based Precautions

Precautions should be taken based on the potential means of transmission, such as contact, droplet, or airborne.

Contact Precautions

Contact precautions are either direct or indirect. Direct would involve a healthcare practitioner who has direct contact with blood or other potentially infectious material. An indirect contact would involve a healthcare practitioner having contact with a contaminated surface such as medical equipment or surfaces in patient care areas. Examples of common pathogens (bacteria) that necessitate contact precautions would include the following:

- Methicillin-resistant *Staphylococcus aureus* (MRSA)
- Vancomycin-resistant enterococcus (VRE)
- *Clostridium difficile* (C. diff)

Gloves and gowns are the minimum required PPE for contact precautions. According to the Centers for Disease Control and Prevention, EMS practitioners should wash their hands with soap and water or use an alcohol-based hand scrub at the following times:

- Prior to touching a patient
- Prior to completing an aseptic treatment or handling invasive medical devices
- Prior to moving from a soiled site to a clean site on the body of the same patient
- After management of a patient or touching their immediate environment
- After contact with blood or body fluids and contaminated areas
- After glove removal

Droplet Precautions

Prevention of transmission by respiratory droplets is referred to as droplet precautions. These respiratory droplets are generated when an infected patient coughs, sneezes, or talks. They are also common during certain procedures such as intubation, cardiopulmonary resuscitation (CPR), or cough induction (i.e., MDI administration). Because the droplets are larger in size, they typically fall with 6 feet of the patient, thus the "social distancing" we have come to know from the

COVID-19 pandemic. Common pathogens that have been generally classified as requiring droplet precautions include the following:

- Pertussis
- Influenza
- Adenovirus
- Rhinovirus
- SARS-CoV-1 and SARS-CoV-2
- Group A *Streptococcus*
- Bacterial meningitis

Medical (surgical/procedure) masks and eye protection are required in addition to the PPE included in contact precautions when treating a patient you suspect may have a disease spread by respiratory droplets.

Airborne Precautions

Airborne precautions are intended to prevent transmission by small respiratory droplets, which can be spread over long distances without direct face-to-face contact. Because these particles are so small, they can be "lofted" in air currents for a long time and be carried over a significant distance. Examples of airborne diseases include the following:

- Tuberculosis (TB)
- Measles
- Varicella-zoster virus, which causes chickenpox and shingles

These type of precautions call for the most PPE and for an airborne isolation room in the hospital. Airborne isolation rooms are negative airflow rooms where fresh air is constantly drawn into the room so airborne particles cannot leave the room. The ambulance environment presents a unique hazard when dealing with airborne isolation patients. The following are some actions that can help limit their spread:

- Sealing off the cab of the ambulance
- Turning on the blower in the front of the ambulance (not on recirculation mode)
- Turning on the exhaust fan in the patient compartment

Aeroso-Generating Procedures

Aerosol-generating procedures should be avoided when possible if you are caring for an infectious patient. The following are procedures that, when performed, generate a fine mist of particles that require airborne precautions:

- Open suctioning of airways
- CPR
- Intubation/extubation
- Noninvasive ventilation (BiPAP, CPAP)

- Manual ventilation (BVM)
- Bronchoscopy
- Nebulizer administration
- High-flow oxygen delivery

If these procedures need to be performed, utilize an airborne isolation room if available. If not available, perform them outside of the transport vehicle. If that is not an option, perform the procedure with doors open and exhaust vents on (while stopped, of course). If stopping is not an option, ensure that the exhaust vents are on high in the patient compartment.

Bloodborne Pathogens

The most common bloodborne pathogens are HIV, hepatitis B virus (HBV), and hepatitis C virus (HCV). The federal OSHA regulations on bloodborne pathogens protection are 29 CFR 1920.1030. The standards include sections on sharps safety, exposure control, hepatitis B vaccination, and requirements for employers to maintain a sharps injury log.

Personal Protective Equipment Considerations

An essential component of utilizing PPE is the consistent use of proper hand hygiene. Ensuring proper hand hygiene before and after the application of all PPE will diminish the opportunity for the inadvertent exposure via the mucous membranes, such as rubbing tired eyes with your hands. Remember, the use of equipment does not replace basic hygiene measures such as hand washing.

PPE is used to protect EMS practitioners and patients by preventing potentially infectious microorganisms from contaminating your hands, eyes, and clothing and being transmitted to others. PPE reduces, but does not completely eliminate, the possibility of acquiring an infection. PPE is only effective if used correctly. The purpose of PPE is to create a barrier between the patient and the EMS practitioner.

For EMS practitioners, PPE includes any combination of nonsterile medical examination gloves; eyewear such as goggles, face shields, or safety glasses; impervious gowns; surgical/procedure masks; and respirators (e.g., N95 masks) that have been fit-tested to ensure adequate protection. Fit-testing is a process to verify the sufficiency of the respirator's seal to the user's face. This can be accomplished in two ways:

- **Qualitative (pass/fail).** The respirator user performs various exercises while exposed to a solution to see if they can taste the solution (either sweet or bitter). If the respirator user does not taste the solution after completion of the fit-test, the user has an adequate seal. If the respirator user tastes the solution during the fit-test, the user has a breach in the seal and the fit-test is failed.

- **Quantitative.** The respirator is attached to a machine that guides the user through various exercises. During the exercises, the machine measures the amount of leak in the seal. Based on the level of the leak, the machine will designate the user as a pass or fail.

EMS practitioners should consider the application of PPE according to the needs of the situation and specifically when there is significant contact with patient or environmental surfaces, a demonstrated need for eye and respiratory protection (as listed earlier in this chapter), or equipment cleaning.

EMS practitioners should not don PPE until they initiate patient care. Premature application of PPE can result in damage to the structural integrity of the PPE as well as environmental contamination transferred to the patient. This damage can create a false sense of protection when in fact there has been a compromise of the PPE to the point of leading to inadvertent inoculation.

PPE should be donned in the following order (1) gown (if needed), (2) mask or respirator (if needed), (3) goggles or face shield (if needed), and (4) gloves (**FIGURE 7-9**). Alcohol-based hand sanitizers can be used as a temporary measure, but soap and water is still the ideal method.

Stay in the Field

It is important to remember that PPE, particularly the examination gloves, will begin to deteriorate once produced. Many factors can accelerate this process. How the gloves and masks are stored within the station and on the apparatus will impact the speed of degradation.

Premature application of PPE can also result in a reduction in the structural integrity of the material. Opening doors and cabinets and maneuvering through a residence will provide opportunities for PPE to be torn, ripped, or otherwise damaged before making patient contact. Some of the degradation may be so minimal that it is not visible, yet it may provide a portal for body fluids to make contact with the EMS practitioner's skin.

Once EMS practitioners have completed patient care, they should properly remove their PPE, with attention to preventing inadvertent cross-contamination. The order is (1) gloves, (2) goggles or face shield, (3) gown, (4) mask or respirator, then hand washing (**FIGURE 7-10**). The PPE should be placed in the appropriate container for disposal. After the removal of all of the PPE, appropriate hand hygiene should be initiated using soap and water or hand rubbing with an alcohol-containing hand cleaner.

Infection Prevention

Utilize the information provided by dispatch to identify patients with symptoms of potentially highly infectious disorders. Maintain a heightened awareness for the potential to interact with patients with new and drug-resistant organisms. Limit the number of personnel who have initial contact with a patient by conducting the "view from the door" to determine the need for multiple practitioners. Should such an impression not be clear, only one EMS practitioner, wearing the appropriate PPE, should make contact and conduct the patient assessment. Be sure to obtain a thorough travel history that covers the past month. Ask the patient about any recent domestic and international travel.

Wear the appropriate level of PPE based on the mode of transmission of the suspect agent. Provide surgical masks to all patients with symptoms of a respiratory illness who can tolerate its placement. Conduct active surveillance for infected sores, ulcers, lesions, and drainage. Cover openings/sores that have drainage. Use contact precautions during close patient contact and wear gloves, gown, and mask to prevent contact contamination on your clothing. Ensure the patient is "wrapped in linen" prior to being moved to minimize environmental contamination. Be sure to confirm that the hospital or other receiving facility has been notified of the possibility of an infectious disease so they can prepare appropriately for your arrival.

Perform thorough cleaning of all equipment that had contact with the patient or the environmental surfaces of the patient's room/home. Ensure that all disinfecting agents are properly approved for use against the suspected pathogen. If you have any questions, check with your agency's medical director.

Dealing With Exposure

It is hoped that most EMS practitioners will go their entire career without experiencing an occupational exposure to an infectious disease. However, even a solid awareness of the potential for infection may not be

SEQUENCE FOR PUTTING ON PERSONAL PROTECTIVE EQUIPMENT (PPE)

The type of PPE used will vary based on the level of precautions required, such as standard and contact, droplet or airborne infection isolation precautions. The procedure for putting on and removing PPE should be tailored to the specific type of PPE.

1. GOWN

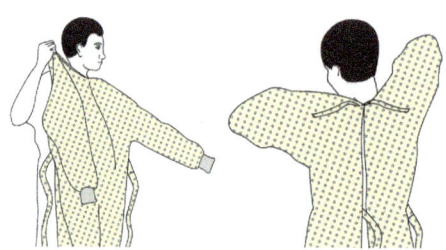

- Fully cover torso from neck to knees, arms to end of wrists, and wrap around the back
- Fasten in back of neck and waist

2. MASK OR RESPIRATOR

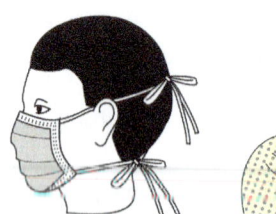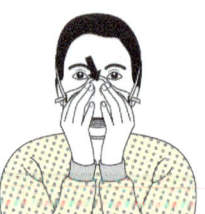

- Secure ties or elastic bands at middle of head and neck
- Fit flexible band to nose bridge
- Fit snug to face and below chin
- Fit-check respirator

3. GOGGLES OR FACE SHIELD

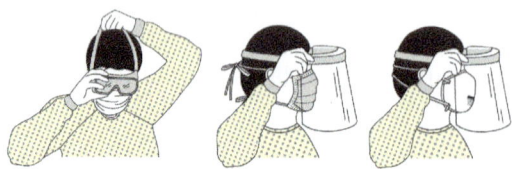

- Place over face and eyes and adjust to fit

4. GLOVES

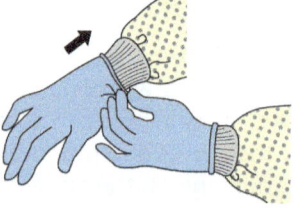

- Extend to cover wrist of isolation gown

USE SAFE WORK PRACTICES TO PROTECT YOURSELF AND LIMIT THE SPREAD OF CONTAMINATION

- Keep hands away from face
- Limit surfaces touched
- Change gloves when torn or heavily contaminated
- Perform hand hygiene

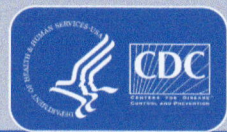

FIGURE 7-9 The sequence for donning PPE.

Courtesy of the Centers for Disease Control and Prevention. Reference to specific commercial products, manufacturers, companies, or trademarks does not constitute its endorsement or recommendation by the U.S. Government, Department of Health and Human Services, or Centers for Disease Control and Prevention. Available free of charge at https://www.cdc.gov/hai/pdfs/ppe/PPE-Sequence.pdf.

HOW TO SAFELY REMOVE PERSONAL PROTECTIVE EQUIPMENT (PPE) EXAMPLE 1

There are a variety of ways to safely remove PPE without contaminating your clothing, skin, or mucous membranes with potentially infectious materials. Here is one example. **Remove all PPE before exiting the patient room** except a respirator, if worn. Remove the respirator **after** leaving the patient room and closing the door. Remove PPE in the following sequence:

1. GLOVES

- Outside of gloves are contaminated!
- If your hands get contaminated during glove removal, immediately wash your hands or use an alcohol-based hand sanitizer
- Using a gloved hand, grasp the palm area of the other gloved hand and peel off first glove
- Hold removed glove in gloved hand
- Slide fingers of ungloved hand under remaining glove at wrist and peel off second glove over first glove
- Discard gloves in a waste container

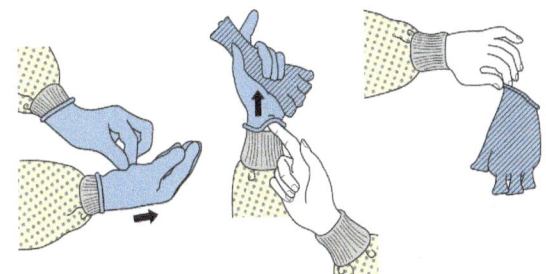

2. GOGGLES OR FACE SHIELD

- Outside of goggles or face shield are contaminated!
- If your hands get contaminated during goggle or face shield removal, immediately wash your hands or use an alcohol-based hand sanitizer
- Remove goggles or face shield from the back by lifting head band or ear pieces
- If the item is reusable, place in designated receptacle for reprocessing. Otherwise, discard in a waste container

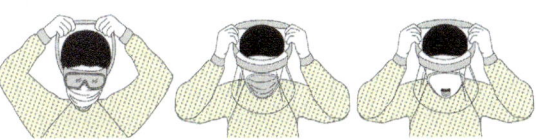

3. GOWN

- Gown front and sleeves are contaminated!
- If your hands get contaminated during gown removal, immediately wash your hands or use an alcohol-based hand sanitizer
- Unfasten gown ties, taking care that sleeves don't contact your body when reaching for ties
- Pull gown away from neck and shoulders, touching inside of gown only
- Turn gown inside out
- Fold or roll into a bundle and discard in a waste container

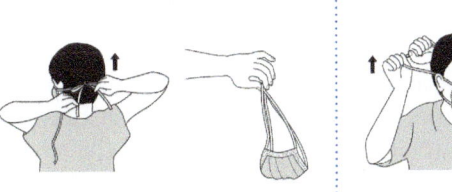

4. MASK OR RESPIRATOR

- Front of mask/respirator is contaminated — DO NOT TOUCH!
- If your hands get contaminated during mask/respirator removal, immediately wash your hands or use an alcohol-based hand sanitizer
- Grasp bottom ties or elastics of the mask/respirator, then the ones at the top, and remove without touching the front
- Discard in a waste container

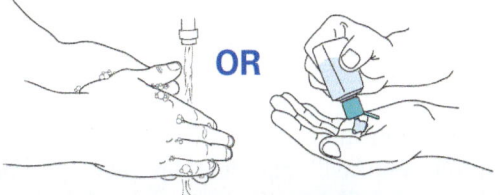

5. WASH HANDS OR USE AN ALCOHOL-BASED HAND SANITIZER IMMEDIATELY AFTER REMOVING ALL PPE

OR

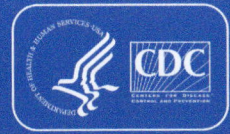

PERFORM HAND HYGIENE BETWEEN STEPS IF HANDS BECOME CONTAMINATED AND IMMEDIATELY AFTER REMOVING ALL PPE

FIGURE 7-10 How to safely remove PPE.

Courtesy of the Centers for Disease Control and Prevention. Reference to specific commercial products, manufacturers, companies, or trademarks does not constitute its endorsement or recommendation by the U.S. Government, Department of Health and Human Services, or Centers for Disease Control and Prevention. Available free of charge at https://www.cdc.gov/hai/pdfs/ppe/PPE-Sequence.pdf.

enough to prevent an EMS practitioner from experiencing such an exposure.

Contact with an infectious agent in and of itself does not result in the development of an infection. To become infected requires an appropriate portal of entry, an adequate amount of the infectious agent, and a susceptible host. For bloodborne pathogen exposures, the transmission risk increases if the injury is deep, if there is evidence of visible blood on the device, if the device was placed in a vein or artery, and if the source patient has indication of a high viral load of the infectious organism.

Regardless of the degree or significance of the exposure, the importance of rapid action in the event of potential exposure cannot be overemphasized. Should evaluation of the exposure indicate that postexposure prophylaxis (PEP) is warranted, such PEP needs to be initiated within hours. For potential HIV infection, the sooner prophylaxis is initiated the better, as the PEP becomes less effective 24 to 36 hours after the exposure. Should the source patient later be found to be negative, PEP can be discontinued.

For those who are unvaccinated or nonresponders to the hepatitis B vaccine, hepatitis B immunoglobulin (HBIG) must be administered within 7 days of the exposure, preferably within 24 hours. If the source patient is hepatitis C positive, there is currently no PEP treatment, and ongoing monitoring and follow-up are essential.

It can be more difficult to determine whether an EMS practitioner has been exposed to a respiratory disease such as meningitis, tuberculosis, or pertussis. Even with a suspicion at the time of patient contact, testing and follow-up will take time. Frequently, exposure is not known until later, because materials from the source patient must be cultured to see if an organism can be grown.

Additionally, special situations may prolong the investigation and final disease determination of the source patient. Examples of such situations include patients who are unconscious, unwilling to consent to testing, or pronounced dead on-scene or shortly after arrival at a medical facility; exposures to an unknown source due to improperly discarded contaminated medical sharps; and events that occur off-duty.

Insect infestations usually do not require postexposure treatment. If exposure to scabies is significant, treatment with a miticidal medication that kills the scabies mite can be considered.

Needlestick Injuries and Safety Needle Systems

One of the greatest risks for acquiring an occupational exposure is through a contaminated needle or other medical sharps. A study by Alhazmi et al. indicated that around 18% of surveyed EMS practitioners reported a needlestick injury (NSI) in the preceding 12 months. Of this group who reported an NSI, there were significant correlations to age, experience, and level of certification, as demonstrated by the following examples:

- 32% of critical care paramedics reported an NSI in the previous 12 months compared to only 27% of paramedics.
- 39% of practitioners with more than 15 years of experience had an NSI in the previous 12 months.
- Half of responders age 60 or older reported a needlestick in the previous 12 months.

The best tool to prevent NSI is to use all engineered sharps safety protections, such as self-sheathing catheters and syringes that cover the needle after use, devices where the needle retracts into the device, and one-time use devices where the needle cannot be redeployed (auto-injectors and lancets). EMS practitioners should ensure proper knowledge on the use and activation of such devices, and the devices should not adversely impact the delivery of patient care or result in EMS practitioners delaying treatment. In addition, no one should attempt to circumvent the intended safety functions of the device. EMS practitioners should ensure that all contaminated medical sharps are properly disposed of into a puncture-resistant container.

Thanks to sharps safety devices, the prevalence of sharps injuries has been gradually decreasing among EMS practitioners.

Cleaning and Disinfection

Equipment and environmental surfaces can provide a mechanism for the spread of infectious diseases from one patient to another and to EMS practitioners. To prevent such mechanisms, it is important to ensure that all equipment that has contact with the patient or the environmental surfaces of the patient's room are properly cleaned and disinfected for the next emergency response. Once all of the associated patient care needs have been addressed, the EMS practitioners should return to the ambulance for cleaning and disinfection.

It is vital that EMS practitioners ensure all disinfecting agents are properly approved for use against the suspected pathogen. For example, the Environmental Protection Agency's List N is a compilation of all disinfectants that are approved for use against the virus that causes COVID-19 (SARS-CoV-2). In addition, pay attention to the surface contact time, as this number is the time that a disinfectant needs to be in contact with the surface to actually "kill" the pathogen. EMS practitioners should refrain from using antiseptic soaps, which only inhibit the growth and development of microorganisms and are typically intended for use on the skin and mucous membranes. Although such antiseptics may be derived from disinfectants, the concentrations are not strong enough to adequately eradicate the organism. Currently, approved disinfectants are adequate in the cleaning and disinfection of the usually encountered organisms. Special cleaning and disinfection is not warranted unless specific recommendations are issued for newly emerging or resistant strains of organisms.

Before commencing with cleaning and disinfection, EMS practitioners should don the appropriate PPE such as gloves, mask, and eyewear to minimize contact with dispersed contaminated materials and potential inadvertent exposure. EMS practitioners should consider cleaning with disposable towels to minimize cross-contamination and laundering issues.

Using approved cleaning and disinfection agent(s), EMS practitioners should wipe down the stretcher frame, mattress, handrails, and any other potentially contaminated stretcher mechanisms. EMS practitioners should make sure they remove all organic material such as blood, other body fluids, and dirt from the equipment. All patient care equipment used on the patient should be thoroughly cleaned before being placed back into the ambulance. Once the equipment has been adequately and totally cleaned, a disinfectant in the appropriate concentration and for the specified contact time should be applied and allowed to air dry.

After cleaning the equipment and removing all PPE, the EMS practitioner should initiate appropriate hand hygiene once again with an alcohol-containing hand cleaner. Only after this cleaning are EMS practitioners once again ready for additional ambulance responses.

CHAPTER WRAP-UP

- Injury prevention begins prior to the shift.
- Use lift assist teams when available.
- Prepare the patient compartment so that seat belts can be used by practitioners.
- Utilize proper PPE based on the pathogen of concern.
- Don and doff PPE properly.
- Provide masks to patients to ensure source control.

SUMMARY

- To prevent both the cumulative effects and immediate, catastrophic effects of lifting, EMS practitioners should minimize both the load and the number of times that they lift.

- In addition to physical injury, unsafe patient handling may cause discomfort and worsen the patient's condition.

- Back injuries have reached epidemic levels in EMS. Back injuries generate both direct and indirect costs to the injured EMS practitioner.

- Although lifting patients cannot be completely avoided, EMS practitioners can identify lifting situations with higher risks and use task-specific patient-handling equipment with proper body mechanics to minimize the effects of lifting on the body.

- Because injuries can occur during routine lifts, EMS practitioners must practice situational awareness and approach each lift as a potential source of injury.

- Safe patient movement combines evidence-based practices and common sense. Evidence-based practices include:
  - Minimizing manual patient handling

(continued)

SUMMARY (continued)

- Utilizing lift assist/lift teams
- Employing patient and environment assessment strategies
- Utilizing patient-handling equipment and devices
- Training and retraining on techniques and equipment use

■ Before lifting a patient, EMS practitioners should evaluate both the patient and the environment to determine how the patient's condition and the environment will impact the ability of the EMS practitioners to move the patient safely.

■ The EMS practitioner must be familiar with the normal functionality of all equipment and immediately report any concerns.

■ Maintain a heightened awareness of the potential for interface with patients with new and resistant organisms.

■ Limit the number of personnel who have initial contact with the patient by conducting the "view from the door." Should such an impression not be clearly evident, only one responder, in the appropriate PPE, should make patient contact and conduct the initial patient assessment.

■ Obtain a thorough travel history that covers the past month.

■ Wear the appropriate level of PPE based on the mode of transmission of the suspect agent.

■ Where respiratory vectors are considered, employ PPE in accordance with airborne and droplet precautions.

■ Provide surgical masks to all patients with symptoms of a respiratory illness who can tolerate their placement.

■ Ensure that contact precautions are used during close patient contact. Gowns and masks must be worn along with gloves to prevent contact contamination on clothing.

■ Confirm that the hospital or other receiving facilities have been notified of the possibility of an infectious disease.

■ Perform thorough cleaning of all equipment that had contact with the patient or the environmental surfaces of the patient's room.

■ Ensure safe and prompt usage of an engineered needle system and proper sharps disposal.

GLOSSARY

cachectic Possessing an appearance of wasting away.

direct costs Those costs commonly associated with out-of-pocket payments. They include payments to physicians, rehabilitation professionals, insurance carriers, and attorneys.

engineering controls Changes made to the work environment through the use of equipment to avoid work-related injury (e.g., specialty stretchers, lateral transfer aids).

indirect costs Costs related to injury that are not covered by insurance. For example, lost productivity.

lift assist team A team utilized to help EMS practitioners with patient lifting, it can be made up of additional responders on the scene, hospital staff, or another ambulance crew called in as backup.

safe patient movement behaviors These behaviors involve movement actions selected by the EMS practitioner that minimize the risk of injury to patients, practitioners, and bystanders during patient movement events.

REFERENCES

Alhazmi RA, Parker RD, Wen S. Needlestick injuries among emergency medical services providers in urban and rural areas. *J Community Health*. 2018;43(3):518-523. doi:10.1007/s10900-017-0446-0

Association for Professionals in Infection Control and Epidemiology. *Guide to Infection Prevention in Emergency Medical Services*. Washington, DC: APIC; 2013.

Austin City Council. Employee safety. *EMS Audit*. 2001;4:50-51.

Centers for Disease Control and Prevention. Hand hygiene guidance. https://www.cdc.gov/handhygiene/providers/guideline.html

Centers for Disease Control and Prevention. Immunization of health-care personnel: recommendations of the Advisory Committee on Immunization Practices (ACIP). *MMWR*. 2011;60(RR07):1-45.

Centers for Disease Control and Prevention. Recommendations for preventing transmission of human immunodeficiency virus and hepatitis B virus to patients during exposure-prone invasive procedures. *MMWR*. 1991;40(RR08):1-9.

Centers for Disease Control and Prevention. Sequence for Putting on Personal Protective Equipment (PPE). Published 2014. https://www.cdc.gov/hai/pdfs/ppe/ppe-sequence.pdf

Centers for Disease Control and Prevention. Updated U.S. Public Health Service guidelines for the management of occupational exposures to HBV, HCV, and HIV and recommendations for postexposure prophylaxis. *MMWR*. 2001; 50(RR11);1-42.

Centers for Disease Control and Prevention. Workplace safety & health topics: emergency medical services workers: injury and illness data. Published 2012. https://www.cdc.gov/niosh/topics/ems/data.html

de Castro AB. Handle with care: the American Nurses Association's campaign to address work-related musculoskeletal disorders. *Online J Issues Nurs*. 2004;25(6):357.

Fass B. Medics are not disposable: injury prevention strategies. [PowerPoint presentation]. *Fit Responder*. 2009.

Feldstein A, Valanis B, Vollmer W, Stevens N, Overton C. The back injury and prevention project pilot study assessing the effectiveness of back attack: an injury prevention program among nurses, aides, and orderlies. *J Occup Med*. 1993;35:114-120.

Joyce MP, Kuhar D, Brooks JT. Occupational acquired HIV infection among health care workers–United States, 1985–2013. *MMWR*. 2014;63:1245-1246.

Lessa FC, Mu Y, Bamberg WM, et al. Burden of *Clostridium difficile* infection in the United States. *N Engl J Med*. 2015;372:825-834.

National Association of Emergency Medical Technicians. EMS fitness. Accessed December 8, 2021. https://www.naemt.org/initiatives/health

Occupational Safety and Health Administration. OSHA procedures for safe weight limits when manually lifting. Accessed December 8, 2021. https://www.osha.gov/laws-regs/standardinterpretations/2013-06-04-0

Oregon Occupational Safety and Health Administration. Firefighter and emergency medical services ergonomics curriculum. Oregon OSHA Consultative Services. Published 2008. https://osha.oregon.gov/edu/grants/train/Documents/Firefighter-and-Emergency-Medical-Services-Ergonomics-Curriculum.pdf

Reichard AA, Marsh SM, Tonozzi TR, Konda S, Gormley MA. Occupational injuries and exposures among emergency medical services workers. *Prehosp Emerg Care*. 2017;21(4):420-431. doi:10.1080/10903127.2016.1274350

Smith N. A National Perspective on Ambulance Crashes and Safety Guidance from the National Highway Traffic Safety Administration on Ambulance Safety for Patients and Providers. Published September 2015. https://www.ems.gov/pdf/EMSWorldAmbulanceCrashArticlesSept2015.pdf

Sternbach RA. Survey of pain in the United States: Nuprin pain report. *Clin J Pain*. 1986;2(1):49-53.

Studnek JR, Ferketich A, Crawford JM. On the job illness and injury resulting in lost work time among a national cohort of emergency medical services professionals. *Am J Ind Med*. 2007;50(12):921-931.

Triano J. Ergonomics of the office and workplace: an overview. *Spine Health*. Published September 26, 2006. Accessed December 8, 2021. https://www.spine-health.com/wellness/ergonomics/ergonomics-office-and-workplace-overview

U.S. Department of Labor, Bureau of Labor Statistics. Employer-Reported Workplace Injuries and Illnesses—2015. Published 2016. Accessed December 8, 2021. https://www.bls.gov/news.release/pdf/osh.pdf

U.S. Department of Labor, Bureau of Labor Statistics. Table R98. Incidence rates for nonfatal occupational injuries and illnesses involving days away from work per 10,000 full-time workers by occupation and selected nature of injury or illness, private industry, 2019. Accessed December 8, 2021. https://www.bls.gov/iif/oshwc/osh/case/cd_r98_2019.htm

Willis MT. Compensation worsens back pain. ABCNews.com. Published January 6, 2006. Accessed December 8, 2021. https://abcnews.go.com/Health/PainManagement/story?id=117092&page=2

CHAPTER 8

Personal Health

LESSON OBJECTIVES

- Identify stressors experienced by EMS personnel.
- Discuss resilience.
- Recognize the impact of stress on a person's mental and physical health.
- Develop an effective fatigue management plan.
- Demonstrate physical fitness techniques.
- Recognize methods for effective hydration and healthy eating.

Scenario

Your kids don't want to go to school today, you can't find your keys, you have no cash, and your significant other took the ATM card. You are now 15 minutes late leaving for work. Your uniform shirt is in the dryer and still damp. If you are late to work one more time, you will get a written reprimand, which will decrease your merit increase and limit your chances for promotion. But you don't hit any red lights, and you make it to work with 3 minutes to spare.

Your regular partner has called in sick, so you'll be working your 12-hour shift with someone you don't particularly like. The ambulance has not been disinfected and is stocked incompletely. Before you can clean the unit and properly restock it, you are called to the scene of a pediatric trauma code, the result of child abuse. You are unable to successfully intubate the child, and the intraosseous supplies are missing. Upon your arrival at the hospital, the emergency department physician is angry about your performance.

1. How many of these events would be stressors for you?
2. How can you keep these events from happening?
3. What strategies do you have in place to help you cope with stressful events?

Introduction

Personal health requires that you be both physically and mentally prepared to deal with the daily issues that life and the job throw at you. This chapter will introduce you to the tools to help you achieve optimal states of physical and mental readiness, as well as information to help you deal with events and conditions that may impair you physically and mentally. Clearly, it is impossible to remove all stressors from your life, but adequate physical and mental preparation can help minimize their impact on you.

To address the problems related to personal health and safety in emergency medical services (EMS), we must first acknowledge that a problem exists. EMS practitioners can experience emotional, physical, and/or psychological stress from their work or home life. Increased levels of stress and injuries on the job can lead to depression, burnout, job loss, and suicide. In fact, EMS practitioners are 10 times more likely to contemplate suicide than the general population. They are 13 times more likely to attempt suicide than the general population. EMS personnel also face health and wellness challenges. They are more likely to miss work due to a work-related injury than police or fire department personnel. In 2009, a study reported that 75% of EMS and fire department personnel were either overweight or obese. Conditions such as sleep apnea, insomnia, and circadian rhythm sleep–wake conditions have demonstrated severe health effects on patients. The circadian rhythm sleep–wake conditions have a significant impact on prehospital professionals due to 24-hour shift work and the relentless waking up to respond to emergency calls.

Stressors in EMS

Stress is considered physical, chemical, or emotional factors that cause physical or psychological tension. Not all stress is bad. In fact, stress can be thought of as occurring along a continuum (**FIGURE 8-1**). **Eustress** is considered positive, beneficial short-term stress. With eustress, psychological balance is restored when a person sees that he or she is capable of tackling life's happy challenges, such as receiving a promotion, getting married, buying a home, having a child, or traveling. In EMS, a good example would be your agency receiving new, updated equipment that you need to learn how to use safely.

Negative stress is distress. **Distress**, as in the term "distressing," disrupts a person's psychological balance

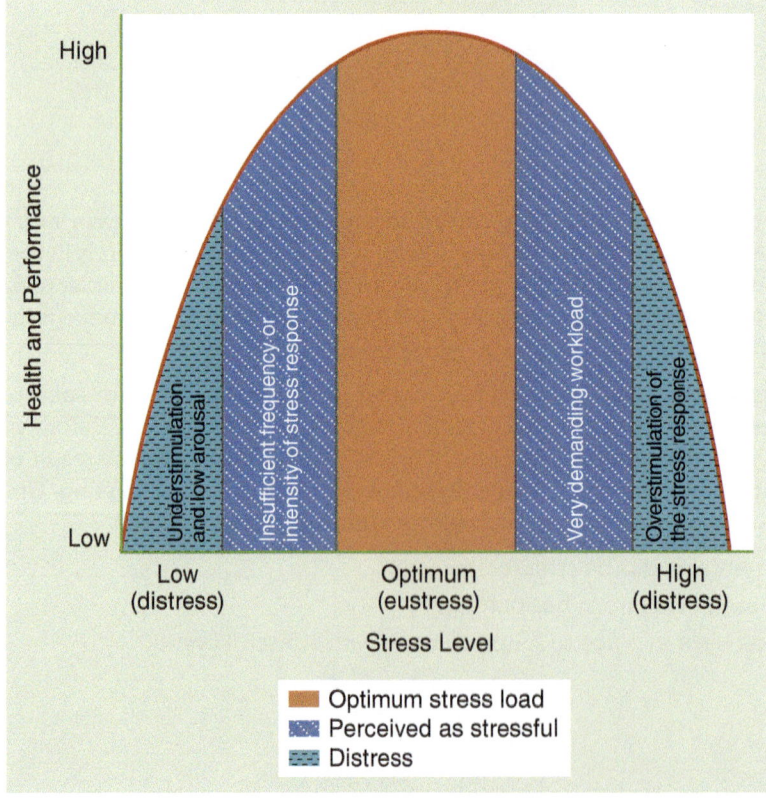

FIGURE 8-1 The continuum of stress.

Reproduced from Quick JC, Quick JD, Nelson DL, Hurrell JJ. *Preventive Stress Management in Organizations*. American Psychological Association; 1997:22.

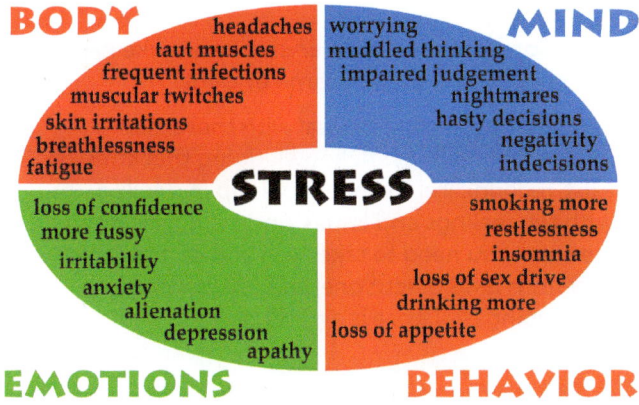

FIGURE 8-2 Optimal mental health is achieved through a balance of work and life outside of work.

© desdemona72/Shutterstock.

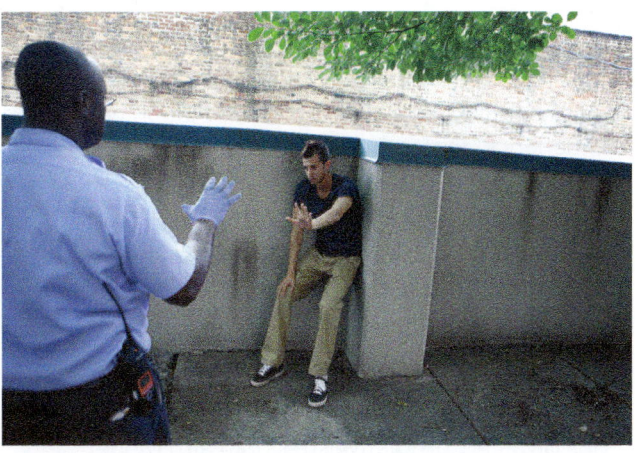

FIGURE 8-3 EMS is filled with daily stressors, from rotating schedules, to mandated overtime, to angry patients.

© Jones & Bartlett Learning. Courtesy of MIEMSS.

and can overwhelm him or her physically and mentally. Examples of situations that lead to distress are the death of a family member, divorce, serious illness or injury of a family member or yourself, financial struggling, conflict in your interpersonal relationships, and challenges with a child's behavior, performance in school, or disability. EMS practitioners may experience distress due to an increased volume in calls, a particularly difficult or tragic call, or a serious disagreement with a coworker or manager.

Mental health impacts relationships, decision-making abilities, and the capacity to handle stress. Optimal mental health is achieved through a balance of work and life outside of work (**FIGURE 8-2**). Maintenance of this balance is called homeostasis. When your expectations and experiences do not match, this balance is disrupted, and stress occurs. The event is relevant to the person involved and can precipitate an emotional response ranging from anxiety to depression. Common physiologic responses to stress include high blood pressure, anxiety, increased heart rate, rapid breathing, headache, insomnia, and depression. Depression is the most common mental health disorder. People with **depression** may experience a lack of interest or pleasure in daily activities, significant weight loss or gain, insomnia or excessive sleeping, lack of energy, inability to concentrate, feelings of worthlessness or excessive guilt, and sometimes recurrent thoughts of death or suicide.

There are both long-term and short-term stressors in EMS. Long-term stressors inherent to EMS include low and/or unpredictable income that can make it difficult to buy a home, complete one's education, achieve family planning, or save for children's college fund, or plan for retirement. The day-to-day (short-term) stressors experienced in the EMS workplace may include rotating schedules, late arrival of next shift relief personnel, shift start unit checks, and rudeness from coworkers, patient reactions, patients' family members, bystanders, and other healthcare workers (**FIGURE 8-3**). On top of this, dispatchers control where you go. EMS practitioners do not control their station and posting locations and whether these facilities consider rest, relaxation, and nourishment. All these issues can add up over time and generate levels of discomfort that are stressful.

You may not immediately see stress-related symptoms in yourself but might find them easy to identify in others. Many of the following symptoms could first be recognized by your coworkers:

- Irritable, aggressive, and impatient. Do you pick fights with patients?
- Overburdened. Do you feel the weight of the world, and is it self-imposed?
- Anxious, nervous or afraid. Are your thoughts racing and you can't switch off?
- Unable to enjoy yourself.
- Depressed and uninterested in life.
- Lost sense of humor or very dark humor.
- Sense of dread.
- Worried about health or complete disrespect for your health.
- Antisocial.
- Alcohol or illicit drug use/abuse.

How often do you experience major and day-to-day stressors on a typical shift? Do you ever feel anxious or depressed? Depression and anxiety are comorbid—in other words, they can happen together. People toss around the words "depression" and "anxiety," but what do they actually mean?

In the Field

It is estimated that 20% of the population will experience depression during their lifetime. About three-quarters of people with depression have recurrent episodes.

Depression can place a strain on relationships, and it can increase the likelihood of divorce. It can also impair an EMS practitioner's ability to interact well with partners, patients, and other healthcare practitioners. People can become depressed after experiencing events such as a loved one's death or a divorce. Cumulative stress can also trigger depression. When depression persists and causes functional impairment in a person's day-to-day activities, it is called reactive depression.

Data from Hasin DS, Sarvet AL, Meyers JL, et al. Epidemiology of adult *DSM-5* major depressive disorder and its specifiers in the United States. JAMA Psychiatry. 2018;75(4):336–346. doi:10.1001/jamapsychiatry.2017.4602

What Can We Do?

As EMS practitioners, the path to reducing the effects of stress includes four important components. First, you need to acknowledge that stressors exist. Identifying when signs and symptoms associated with stress exist is critical to recognizing a need for help. Second, you need to recognize the need for help. Self-awareness is an important part of recognizing when the level of stress is becoming more difficult for an individual to cope with. EMS practitioners should be aware of

Stay in the Field

Anxiety is a vague feeling of dread. Physical, emotional, mental, and behavioral reactions can occur simultaneously. Sensations such as queasiness, dizziness, and feeling like your heart is pounding combine with emotions of tenseness, fear, dread, or panic.

Physical signs and symptoms of anxiety include aches, pains, diarrhea, constipation, increased urinary frequency, changes in carbohydrate metabolism, nausea, dizziness, chest pain, tachycardia, loss of sex drive, frequent colds, and irregular menses. Behavioral signs and symptoms may include changes in eating and sleeping habits accompanied by excessive use of alcohol, tobacco, medications, or illegal drugs. Procrastination and social isolation can occur

in persons with anxiety. Nervous habits like nail biting or pacing may become evident.

What can we do to deal with these clearly unpleasant feelings? Acknowledging that stressors exist, recognizing the need for help in dealing with the feelings and issues, and asking for help are steps you need to take; how you do that will vary from EMS practitioner to EMS practitioner. Developing resilience is a good place to start.

available resources such as employee assistance programs (EAPs), peer support, mental health facilities, and other forms of support in their community (all discussed later in this chapter).

Third, ask for help. Reaching out might seem difficult for a number of reasons. The stigma associated with asking for help continues to be an obstacle to EMS personnel seeking help. Many practitioners feel like they cannot trust their organizational EAP or peers. They may feel that reaching out for help could be seen as a sign of weakness. Many resources exist to assist EMS personnel, such as The Code Green Campaign. Since opening in 2014, The Code Green Campaign has assisted thousands of EMS professionals and first responders through raising mental health awareness. Maintaining mental health resilience has proven to increase a person's quality of life.

People who seek help often report stronger relationships with family and friends. Studies report

Stay in the Field

In 2020, 130 people died from suicide each day (on average) in the United States. It has been said that suicide is "a permanent solution to an impermanent condition." If you suspect that your partner or coworker is feeling overwhelmed by life, has confided having such thoughts, or has expressed them on social media, or if you have had such thoughts, bring a supervisor into your circle of trust. There are resources that can help you, a partner, or a coworker regain balance and a sense of purpose. Another option is to contact a resource directly, such as the National Suicide Prevention Lifeline at 1-800-273-8255 or The Code Green Campaign at 1-888-731-3473. Asking for help or obtaining help is not a sign of weakness or betraying a confidence—it is providing life-saving care.

Data from Centers for Disease Control and Prevention. Facts about suicide. https://www.cdc.gov/suicide/facts/index.html

decreased rates of morbidity from medical disorders and early death, due to seeking mental health care. Reach out and select a mental health provider in your region that advocates for patient-centered care. Finally, the fourth component that can aid EMS personnel in handling stress and improving their quality of life is to develop resilience skills.

Work–Life Balance

Maintaining a work–life balance can be difficult. Your optimal mental health is achieved through a balance of work and life. Mental health is critical in maintaining relationships, decision making, and handling stress. Steps that can be taken to reduce and manage stress in the workplace include the following:

- **Set daily goals that can be easily managed.** Make a list and prioritize it with the most important tasks listed first. Simply crossing goals off a list helps promote a sense of success and control. Goals should be realistic and achievable. Studies show a correlation between stress and control. Stress will be reduced by increasing the amount of control people feel they have over their work.
- **Use your time at work wisely.** Avoid procrastination, as the work will grow in your mind, leading to a feeling of being overwhelmed. Divide larger projects at work into smaller ones. Completing the smaller tasks will provide a sense of accomplishment and continued momentum.
- **Take breaks and reward yourself for completing tasks.** Short breaks will allow you time to clear your mind and prepare yourself to better manage stress.
- **Notify your supervisor if you feel overwhelmed by unnecessary work.**
- **Use your vacation and sick time.** These are provided as part of your compensation package. Vacations have proven to provide a needed recharge from work, and they increase morale and productivity. You do not have to travel to take vacation time. Many people enjoy staying home and touring their region. Some organizations enforce vacation time for employees to ensure practitioners are getting the break their bodies need. Sick time is provided to ensure you stay mentally and physically healthy. Use this time to focus on your health. Healthy employees equal productive employees.
- **Use effective communication.** Notify your supervisor or colleagues when you are feeling overwhelmed. You may find that others feel this way, too. Avoid complaining versus seeking out options. Stress could be reduced by looking at a situation through another perspective.

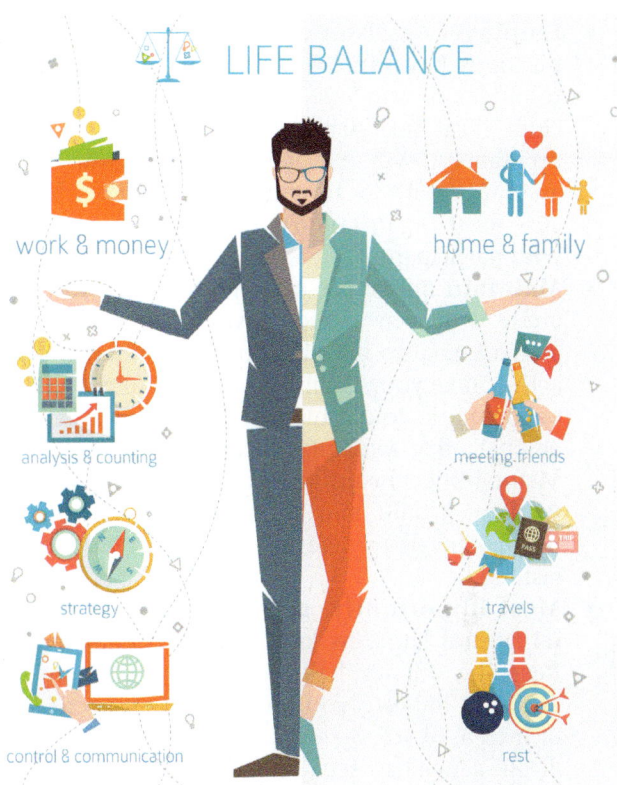

FIGURE 8-4 Optimal mental health is achieved through a balance of work and life.
© Ksyu Deniska/Shutterstock.

- **Maintain a sense of calm and rationality when in a tense position.** Allow others to provide their opinions. Be flexible and compromise. Leave the situation before losing control. Give yourself time to cool down.
- **No one is perfect, so accept that you will make mistakes.** Do the best you can, and know that you are human just like everyone around you (**FIGURE 8-4**).

Steps that can be taken to reduce and manage stress at home include the following:

- **Take time away from work.** Picking up extra shifts or having a second or third job can be nice for the bank account but adds to personal stress. Too much work could lead to burnout. Identify the need for personal time and make it mandatory for yourself.
- **Use your time at home wisely just like at work.** Make a list of home responsibilities and ensure that they are evenly distributed among family members.
- **Learn to say no!** Avoid overscheduling yourself. Looking at a busy calendar adds to your stress.
- **Use your support system.** Family and friends are critical to reducing stress and increasing success at work and home. Support systems are linked to people having an increased immune response, leading to better health.

- **Employee assistance program.** Many organizations have an EAP that provides a variety of resources to employees. These resources may include legal aid, mental health referrals, nutrition programs, travel and gym membership discounts, assistance with locating day care centers, etc. Discuss local organizational EAP program resources with participants.
- **Maintain an active and healthy lifestyle.** Exercise is proven to reduce stress, depression, and anxiety. You do not have to enroll in a gym to be active. Take your family on walks, bike rides, hikes, or to a park. Join athletic leagues such as softball, baseball, flag football, basketball, pickle ball, etc. Maintaining a healthy diet can seem difficult when working a shift and anticipating a call. Prepare healthy meals to take to work rather than eating fast food.
- **Most importantly, get help when you need it!** Do not let stress keep you from enjoying life. Reaching out for help is a sign of strength and does not indicate you are weak. Consistent signs of increased stress should not be avoided and indicate a need to seek help from a mental health professional.

Fitness and Health

Physical fitness is a requirement of being an EMS practitioner. Overall fitness is not determined solely by the amount of weight that a person can lift. An EMS practitioner must be able to bend, twist, reach, and pull repetitively in a manner that hurts neither the EMS practitioner nor the patient (**FIGURE 8-5**). As an EMS

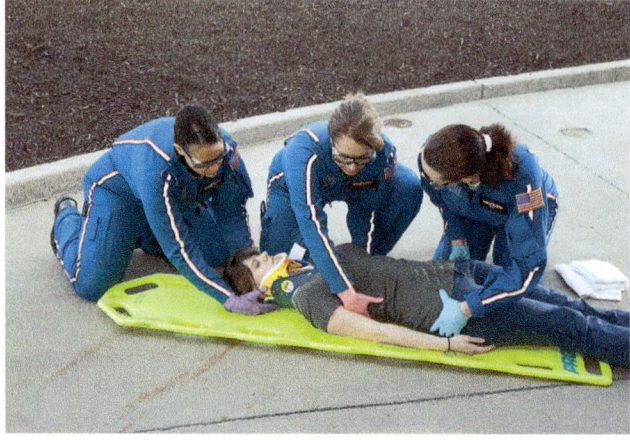

FIGURE 8-5 An EMS practitioner will bend, twist, reach, and pull repetitively throughout the shift.
© National Association of Emergency Medical Technicians (NAEMT).

practitioner, you need to have the functional strength, stability, and mobility to tolerate the daily stresses imposed on your body. Without fitness, your body will not be able to tolerate daily stressors. EMS practitioners often find themselves in unbalanced positions with limited resources.

Fitness is a critical component of overall physical and mental wellness, in addition to being able to meet the physical requirements of the job. Regular physical activity, healthy eating, and stress reduction all improve overall wellness. An essential step in achieving fitness is addressing any body weight issues.

The two most powerful tools in the weight control toolbox are diet and exercise. Let us explore how to use these tools in our daily lives.

Exercise Guidelines

When designing or refining a personal exercise program, it is a good idea to consult with a certified personal trainer to guide you safely to improve mobility, strength, and cardiovascular status. This will help you prevent injuries. In partnership with NAEMT, the American Council on Exercise (ACE) developed "Task Performance and Health Improvement Recommendations for Emergency Medical Services Practitioners." We recommend that you read this document, which can be found at NAEMT.org, on the EMS Fitness page of the Health, Wellness, and Resilience section of the Initiatives tab. This publication is designed to provide general exercise guidelines for EMS practitioners. The ACE program focuses on improving the EMS practitioner's mobility, in addition to strength and cardiovascular training, to prevent injuries that can occur while performing daily activities.

According to Gray Cook, MSPT, OCS, CSCS, the movements performed during daily activities can be broken down into five basic patterns (**FIGURE 8-6**). To avoid injury, ACE recommends that EMS practitioners do the following:

- Perform exercises that train the five basic movement patterns at least 2 days per week.
- Perform moderate-intensity cardiorespiratory physical activity (such walking) 150 minutes per week, *or* perform 75 minutes per week of intense cardiorespiratory physical activity (such as running).

The five basic movement patterns include the following (**FIGURE 8-7**):

- **Bending/raising and lifting/lowering.** Cot movements, standing up from a chair.
- **Single-leg movements.** Stairs and running.
- **Upper body pushing movements.** Transferring a patient or walking while pushing the stretcher.

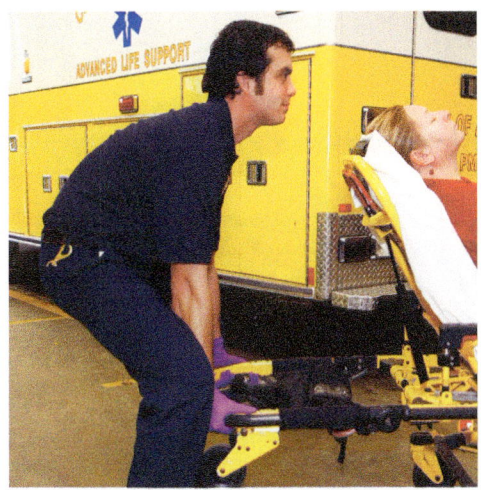

A

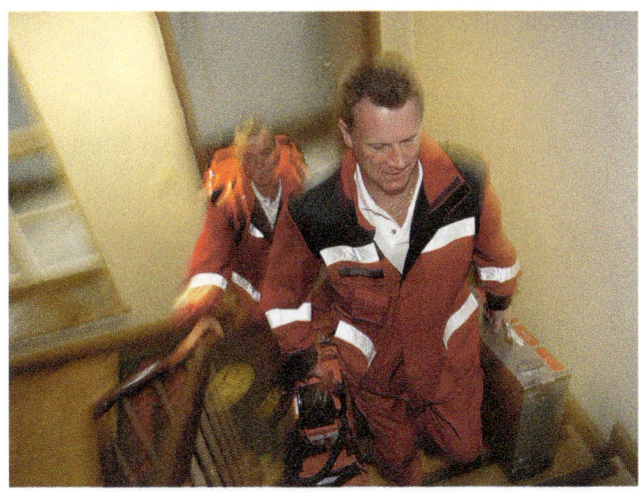

B

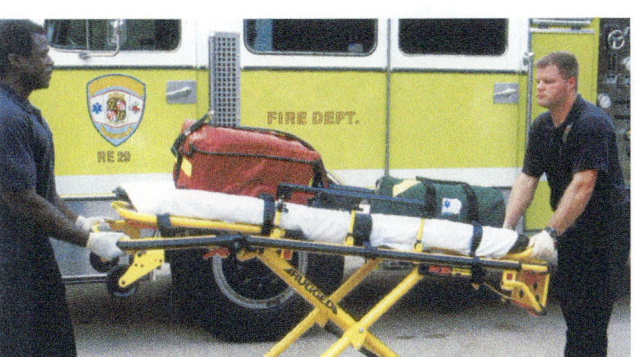

C

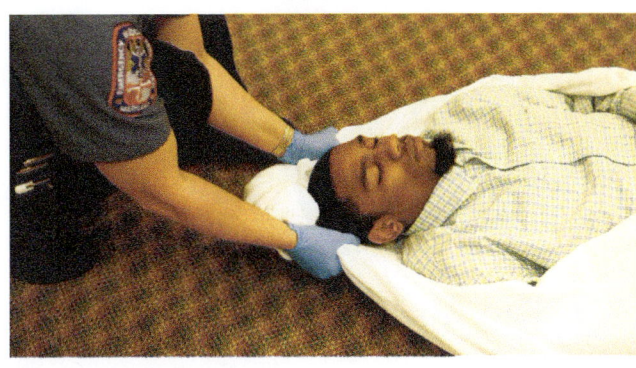

D

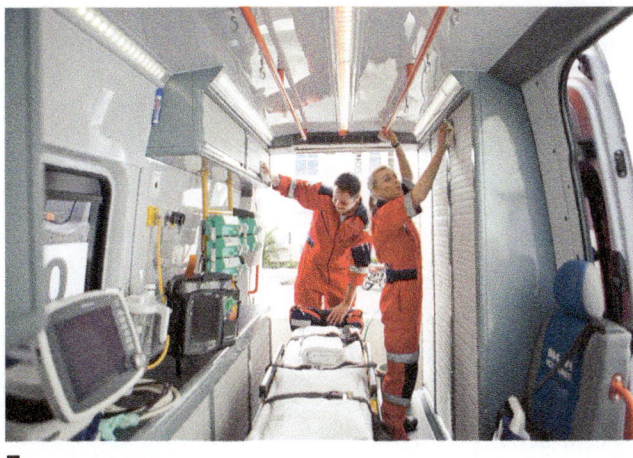

E

FIGURE 8-6 There are five basic movements performed during daily activities. **A.** Bending/raising and lifting/lowering movements. **B.** Single-leg movements. **C.** Upper body pushing movements. **D.** Upper body pulling movements. **E.** Rotational movements.

- **Upper body pulling movements.** Lateral transfer of a patient or removing a patient during an extrication, pulling a stretcher closer toward you.
- **Rotational movements.** Try to limit this movement while holding a weight; use sitting in the patient compartment of an ambulance, reaching for something, twisting from the waist.

Remember that you can be creative and incorporate exercise into your daily routine. Each time you complete a transport, perform one stretch on the back of

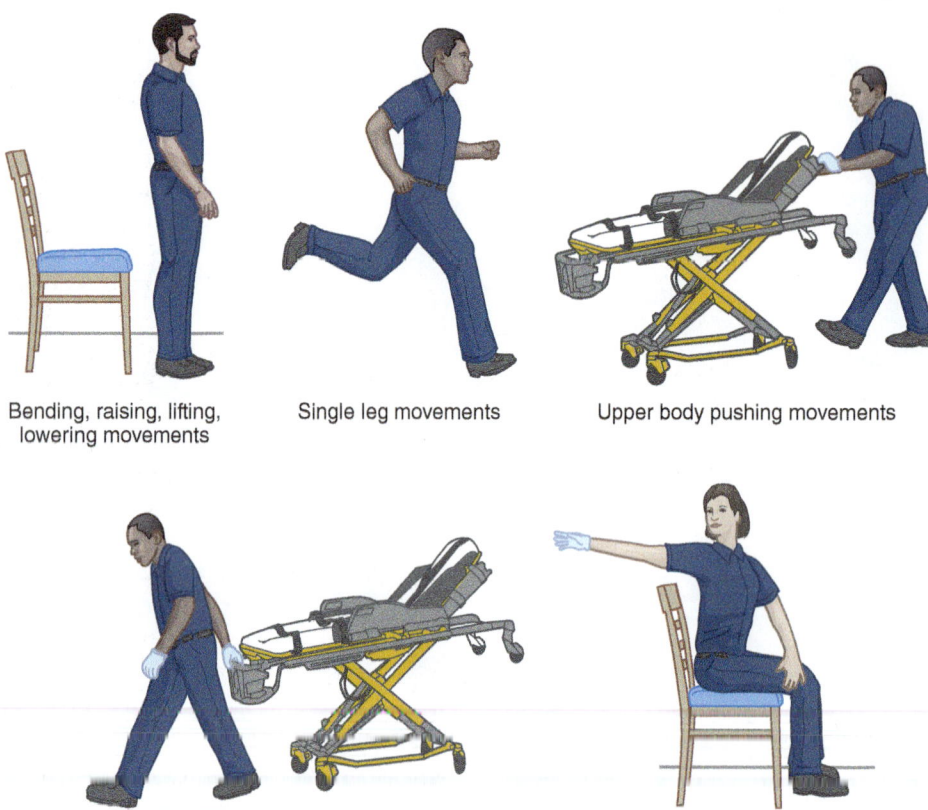

Bending, raising, lifting, lowering movements

Single leg movements

Upper body pushing movements

Upper body pulling movements

Rotational movements

FIGURE 8-7 The five basic movement patterns.
© Jones & Bartlett Learning.

the ambulance (**FIGURE 8-8**). This will keep your body loose and primed for the next call. Simple activities, such as doing step-ups and push-ups on the back of the ambulance between calls, burn calories. Every little bit of exercise adds up!

Avoid Injury and Stay Hydrated

To avoid injury, ACE recommends (1) performing exercises that train the five basic movement patterns at least 2 days per week and (2) performing moderate-intensity cardiorespiratory physical activity such as walking 150 minutes per week or 75 minutes of intense cardiorespiratory physical activity (such as running) per week.

Staying adequately hydrated is essential. Water is the best choice for hydration for the following reasons:

- Helps lubricate the joints
- Helps blood deliver oxygen
- Cushions the brain and spinal cord
- Regulates body temperature
- Flushes out body waste
- Prevents kidney damage

If you wait until you are thirsty or do not need to urinate every 90 minutes, then you are already short of

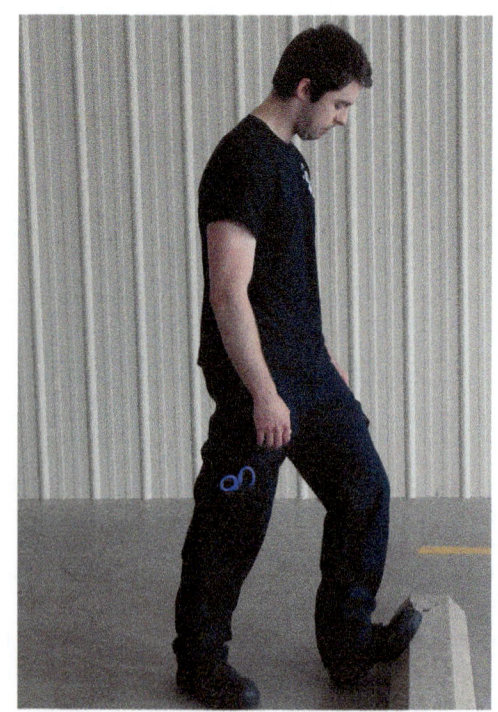

FIGURE 8-8 Stretching between calls will keep you limber and ready.
© Bryan Fass. Used with permission.

water. Dehydration can make EMS practitioners prone to muscle spasms and infections. When working outdoors, especially in high heat, it is easy to underhydrate and become dehydrated. Another good measure of hydration status is that clear urine means adequate hydration, whereas dark or concentrated urine means dehydration.

Poor hydration can be dangerous to your body and brain. Do not fool yourself into drinking sugary drinks in an effort to hydrate. Sugary drinks could lead to dehydration via osmotic diuresis. Studies have shown that people who ingest the artificial sweeteners in "diet" beverages have higher cardiovascular morbidity and mortality than those who do not. Many artificial sweeteners used in these drinks confuse the body and are actually wrapped in fat by the body and stored. Reasons for drinking these beverages are often due to poor planning, lack of storage, and convenience.

Meal Planning

Making healthy food choices is challenging enough when you are at home with a refrigerator full of fresh fruits and vegetables. Obtaining healthy food choices while you are on duty is an even greater challenge. Clearly no single diet plan works for everyone. You must keep track of your intake and modify your diet according to your goals. Eating for "fullness" rather than nutrition leads to increased body fat, sodium, and resting glucose levels and makes people more prone to cancer, cardiovascular disease, and immune system issues. Set yourself up for success by preplanning and bringing healthy meals with you (**FIGURE 8-9**).

Today's education on nutrition suggests eating nutrient-dense foods from the five food groups in the right amounts based on your age, gender, and activity level. For example, a moderately active woman between the ages of 19 and 30 requires around

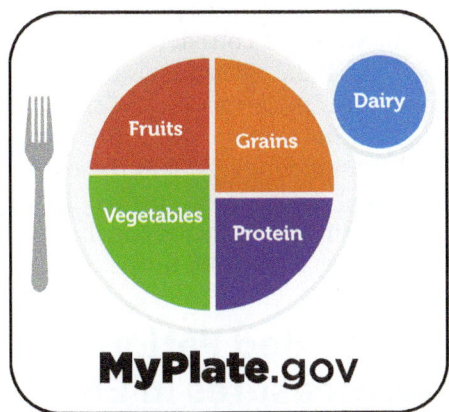

FIGURE 8-9 Helpful information is available at MyPlate and the MyPlate Calorie Counter sites.

Courtesy of the U.S. Department of Agriculture.

2,000 calories per day, whereas a moderately active man requires about 200 calories more.

Regarding the food groups, the current advice is as follows:

- **Fruits.** Eat a variety of fruits; choose fresh, frozen, canned, or dried fruit. Go easy on fruit juices. Read labels; corn syrup should be avoided altogether. Look for products that have no sugar added. (Recommended: 1 cup or 100% fruit juice or ½ cup dried fruit.)
- **Vegetables**. Vary the vegetables you eat; eat more dark green, red, and orange vegetables, as well as dried beans and peas. Half of your plate should be fruits and vegetables. (Recommended: 1 cup raw or cooked vegetables or vegetable juice. Two cups raw leafy greens can substitute for 1 cup vegetables.)
- **Grains.** Make half your grains whole. Whole grains are healthier because they contain important nutrients that reduce the risk of disease. They also contain more protein and more fiber. Consume 3 ounces of whole-grain bread, cereal, crackers, rice, or pasta every day. Look for the word "whole" before the grain name on the list of ingredients. (Recommended: 1 slice of bread, 1 cup of ready-to-eat cereal or ½ cup cooked rice, pasta, or cooked cereal counts as 1 ounce-equivalent.)
- **Protein**. Go lean on protein; choose low-fat or lean meats and poultry. Bake, broil, or grill. Vary your choices with more fish, beans, peas, nuts, and seeds. (Recommended: 1 ounce of meat, poultry, or fish; ¼ cup cooked beans; or 1 egg. 1 tablespoon of peanut butter or ½ ounce of nuts or seeds can be considered as 1 ounce-equivalent.)
- **Dairy.** Eat calcium-rich foods, choosing low-fat or fat-free items. (Recommended: 1 cup of milk, yogurt, or soy milk, or 1½ ounces of natural cheese can be considered as 1 cup.)
- **Fats.** Although not a food group, you should know your fats. Make most fat sources from fish, nuts, and vegetable oils. Limit solid fats like butter, stick margarine, shortening, and lard.

Finally, it is a good idea to check the amount of sodium in canned and prepared foods; choose those with lower amounts. How do you match your diet to the plate? Consider using myplate.gov as a resource to get ideas and strategies for healthy eating. MyPlate Calorie Counter is a useful app for reference. Additional resources are available, such as Apple Watch, FitBit, Google Watch, the MyFitnessPal app, etc.

Sleep and the Brain

Sleep is critical for proper brain function. Throughout the waking hours, the brain collects waste products on the cellular level. While people sleep, the brain processes these waste products and removes them. The lymphatic system mimics the flow of blood in the body and works to remove waste and byproducts. While the body absorbs the good, the lymphatic system removes the bad with one exception, the brain, which does this work itself. This waste removal is achieved via cerebrospinal fluid (CSF). When people sleep, CSF flows throughout the brain to fill the void from missing blood, slightly decreasing the size of the brain. As people cycle through the five sleep stages (about 90 minutes each) the CSF circulates, gently cleansing the brain of toxins. Studies show that CSF flows to the brain during non-rapid eye movement (NREM) sleep to clear toxins linked to neurodegenerative diseases (e.g., Alzheimer disease).

Exhaustion is a major component of burnout. Sleep does not guarantee that you will be rested or relaxed when you awaken; you cannot rely solely on the quality of sleep to ensure adequate rest. "I had 3 hours of good sleep last night" is an illusion of adequacy. If you do not get 7 to 8 hours of sleep every 24 hours, as recommended by the Sleep Foundation, for adults ages 26 to 64 years, you are not meeting your physiologic needs. If you lose 2 hours of sleep per night over 5 consecutive days, you will accumulate a sleep debt of 10 hours. However, you cannot go five or six nights with minimal sleep and make up for it by sleeping 12 hours in one night.

> ### Stay in the Field
>
> Sleep failure has many causes. The following are among the causes of sleep restriction or loss:
>
> - **Job-related.** 24-hour shifts and mandatory overtime.
> - **Personal demands.** "My baby has croup."
> - **Lifestyle choices.** "I don't need to be at work until 0800, so I can stay up until 0200!"
> - **Sleep fragmentation.** Overnight calls.
> - **Disruptions to the body's clock.** Jet lag, night shifts, or alternating day/night shifts.
> - **Use of sedating medication.** Antihistamines or cough suppressants.
> - **Untreated sleep disorders.** Sleep apnea.

Fatigue Management and Sleep Debt

A regular sleep schedule and regular bedtime allow you to recover faster on your days off. Rest, relaxation, and sleep are critical for stress management. Inadequate

sleep could lead to decreased cognitive and psychomotor skills. It may also cause sexual dysfunction, gastrointestinal disturbances, immune system dysfunction, and microsleeps. During microsleeps the eyes close and the mind ceases to be aware of its surroundings.

> ### Stay in the Field
>
> Sleep debt can lead to drowsy driving. Driving is a complex task involving both mental and physical skills. Situational awareness, decision-making abilities, motor control, and reaction time are all impaired in the drowsy driver.

Inadequate sleep leads to sleep debt. **Sleep debt** is the difference between the amount of sleep you get and the amount that your body needs. The Sleep Foundation recommends that people in the 26 to 64 age range get 7 to 9 hours of sleep every 24 hours. If you lose 2 hours of sleep per night over 5 consecutive days, you accumulate sleep debt of 10 hours. However, physiology does not allow people to pay back the sleep debt in a lump sum. Sleep debts impact your behavior and can negatively impact you both physically and mentally by impairing your focus, reflexes, thinking, and social skills. Try to get at least 4 to 5 hours of quality sleep every 24 hours. Interestingly, 3% of the population has a genetic mutation (ADRB1) that allows a person to function on 6 hours or less of sleep. Of course, that 3% of the population cannot all be EMS practitioners!

Shortage of sleep can degrade neurologic response to an extent that mimics alcohol intoxication. Studies show after 17 hours of wakefulness, participants performed as if they had a blood alcohol level of 0.05. At 24 hours without rest, participants operated in much the same manner as someone with a blood alcohol level of 0.10, which is considered legally intoxicated in many regions. If the sleep debt is too great, the body will take measures to correct the deficit in the form of microsleeps. During a **microsleep**, the mind ceases to be aware of its surroundings, and the eyes may close for a short period. Microsleeps may last from a few seconds to a few minutes. A microsleep that occurs while driving could be fatal (**FIGURE 8-10**).

Recommended Fatigue Countermeasures in EMS

At best, countermeasures for drowsy drivers are stopgaps and are no replacement for adequate sleep. A study

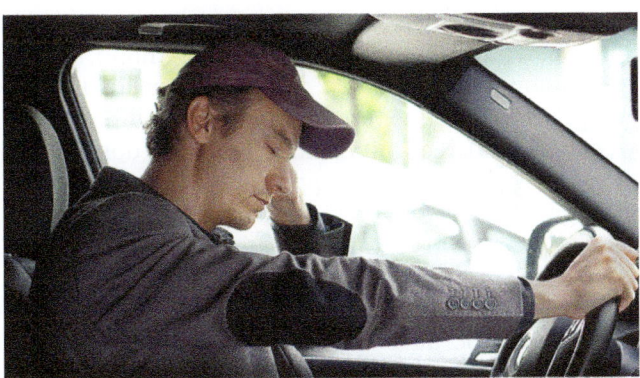

FIGURE 8-10 Microsleeps are one way the body copes with a sleep debt. Microsleeps can be deadly if they occur while a person is behind the wheel.
© StarsStudio/iStockphoto.

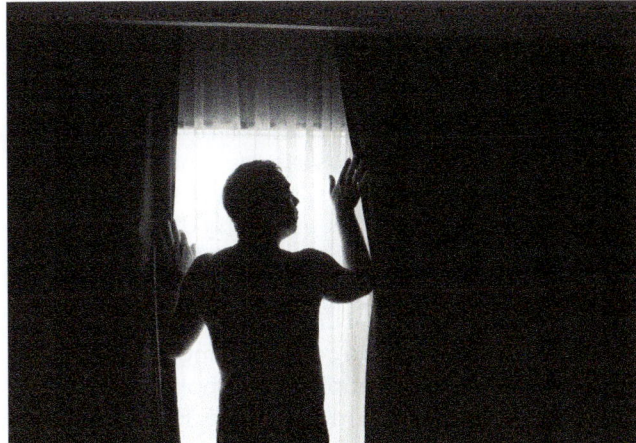

FIGURE 8-11 If you must sleep during the day because of shift work, light-blocking curtains can help create more ideal sleeping conditions.
© Oleg Golovnev/Shutterstock.

supports the following fatigue countermeasures for EMS personnel:

- Allowing crew members to nap when possible and providing an area to rest.
- Caffeine is effective only when it is not used all day, every day. To be most effective, it should only be used when needed.
- Using a pre-, during, and post-shift fatigue assessment tool as part of an overall fatigue management plan.
- Providing education about fatigue, sleep cycles, and the effects that lack of sleep will cause.
- Changing shift lengths, providing adequate time off, expecting downtime prior to shift.
- Following the standards recommended by the Commission on Accreditation of Medical Transport Standards (CAMTS) and Commission on Accreditation of Ambulance Services (CAAS). For example, 10 hours of downtime prior to the start of any shift; a fatigue management plan, with rest periods, for 24-hour shifts; and allowing no crew to be forced to work 4 hours past the end of a 24-hour shift.

Naps can be a helpful way to pay the sleep debt, but naps greater than 45 minutes may risk sleep inertia. Naps of 45 minutes or more, but less than 90 minutes, are like opening a dishwasher mid-cycle; this is where the inertia feeling comes from. Sleep inertia can last up to 20 minutes. Naps of about 30 minutes are preferred. If you are utilizing caffeine as a countermeasure, it takes approximately 30 minutes to take effect. So, you could drink your caffeine, set an alarm for a 30-minute nap, and by the time you wake up your caffeine will be working.

Good Sleep Habits

Good sleep habits are vital to avoid building up sleep debt. Try to maintain a regular sleep schedule at work and at home. Do not read, eat, or watch TV in bed. Do not scroll social media or play video games as these activities "wake up" the brain and make it more difficult to go to sleep. Avoid caffeine and alcohol before bedtime. Don't eat for an hour to an hour and a half before going to bed. Keep your bedroom comfortable by avoiding temperature extremes and bright lights, masking outside noises with "white noise" devices or an electric fan, and making the bedroom as dark as possible by using room-darkening blinds or blackout curtains (**FIGURE 8-11**). Daytime sleepers should silence telephones and related devices.

Resilience

Resilience is the ability to cope with stress and adversity without suffering lasting physical or psychological harm. Some people seem to be able to quickly accept life's challenges and difficulties; however, many EMS practitioners need training to strengthen their resilience skills and to lessen the impact of stressors and trauma that might cause depression, anxiety, post-traumatic stress, or post-traumatic stress disorder (PTSD). Studies show that resilience is not a fixed trait but is a set of skills that can be taught and learned. Resilience skills enable EMS practitioners to adapt and manage both daily stressors and major life events. Resilience does not occur spontaneously, as it requires specific training to develop physical, behavioral, cognitive, and social resilience skills. These skills are enhanced by attitudes, behaviors, and social supports that can be adopted and cultivated.

Stay in the Field

In addition to taking the time to recognize stress in ourselves, it is important to communicate well with and be sensitive to the emotional needs of your coworkers. It is part of the culture of safety to be open about sharing difficulties and identifying the times when stress levels are high. Signs and symptoms of stress that are important to note in ourselves and others include anxiousness, difficulty concentrating, being easily irritated, avoiding people and responsibilities, being quick to anger, overreacting, having fatigue, and exhibiting nervous behaviors such as nail biting, pacing, or teeth grinding. Potential physical manifestations of stress include chest palpitations; headaches; digestive problems; muscle tension and pain; disrupted sleep patterns; hypertension; weight loss or gain; skin problems such as acne, rashes, and hives; and hair loss.

Organizational Attributes Supporting Resilience and Wellness

Just as your organization's leadership is essential in fostering a culture of safety, they also have a key role in supporting resilience and wellness. The workplace is a source of social support, and EMS organizations can and should offer opportunities for connection among employees. Coworkers may also serve as an extended family. This is particularly true in EMS, where teamwork is essential and EMS practitioners form strong bonds as a result of shared experiences, such as saving a life or witnessing death. The opportunity to build friendships at work can contribute to a sense of belonging and a shared mission, and it may offer support in helping to face life's challenges.

Organizations can support good physical health, because physical health is associated with good mental health and resilience. Getting sufficient sleep, nutrition, and exercise can ward off chronic illness, boost one's mood, and protect against depression. People who are physically healthy are better able to face the emotional and psychological challenges of working in EMS. Organizational leadership can establish policies and initiatives that promote healthy lifestyles. Examples include smoking cessation, weight loss programs, opportunities to exercise, and fatigue mitigation. Healthy choices in the vending machines in your station are another example. Does the leadership foster positivity and optimism, which have also been shown

to bolster resilience? The work environment should be one in which employees receive recognition and appreciation for their work. Leadership needs to show employees that they are valued by providing positive feedback and recognition for a job well done. Initiatives should also provide opportunities for peer-to-peer recognition.

Organizations should help their employees adapt to change. Change can be very stressful, whether it is a new company owner or new protocols for performing a procedure. Organizational transparency and a commitment to keeping employees informed will create an environment in which individuals are better able to accept change. Examples of helping employees adapt to change include obtaining employee feedback prior to implementing a change, leading by example, clearly communicating the benefits of the change, and providing adequate training on implementing the change. Progressive organizations empower employees to identify solutions. Research suggests that individuals with strong problem-solving skills tend to be more resilient. Having a sense of control over one's circumstances also boosts resilience. Organizations can challenge employees to make meaningful contributions to the workplace by asking for their input on how to improve working conditions. An empowering organization will make sure employees know how their feedback is incorporated into new policies or procedures.

Why Is Resilience Important?

The fatality rate for EMS practitioners is two and a half times the national average, and EMS practitioners are three times more likely to miss work because of injury. In addition, because of daily exposure to life-threatening and life-ending events, EMS practitioners are more vulnerable to post-traumatic stress disorder, a delayed stress reaction to a traumatic incident. It is estimated that 15% to 20% of EMS practitioners experience PTSD at some point in their career. In addition, PTSD can increase the risk of alcohol or drug abuse and suicide.

How Do We Address the Problem?

There are national and local programs designed to help EMS practitioners to develop or improve their resilience skills. Developing these skills helps prepare a person to respond to stressors with greater resilience. Resilience skills can be thought of like tools in a toolbox—they can be pulled from the toolbox and used as needed.

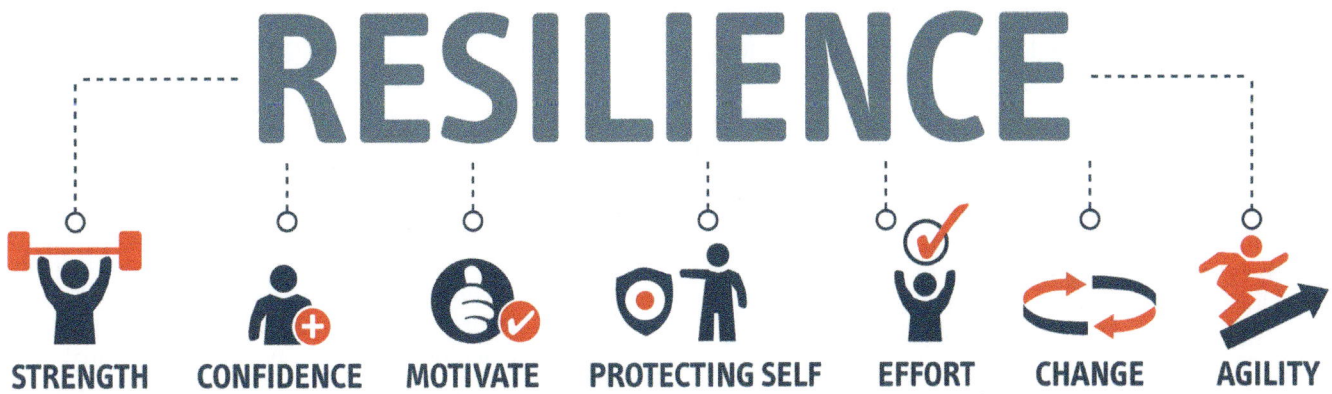

FIGURE 8-12 Skills that should be in your resilience toolbox.

© Trueffelpix/Shutterstock.

What's in the Resilience Toolbox?

The first skills in the resilience toolbox are the physical and behavioral skills that help provide optimal physical health. To cope well, EMS practitioners need to feel well. The skills are goal setting, healthy eating, exercise, sleep, and relaxation. By integrating these physical and behavioral skills, EMS practitioners are better prepared to deal with stress and utilize the more cognitive and socially oriented resilience skills (**FIGURE 8-12**).

The cognitive and social skills address putting situations and feelings into perspective, understanding the fundamentals of your beliefs, understanding your self-defeating thoughts, practicing empathy, coping with your wins and losses, reaching out for support, and accessing social support.

Physical and Behavioral Skills

The balance of resilience tools under the physical and behavioral skills category includes healthy eating, exercise, sleep, and relaxation. When your body is functioning well, you are much more capable of physically and mentally coping with stress.

The physical and behavioral skills build on current baseline measures. Students assess their current physical and behavioral states and identify how a healthier lifestyle could improve these states. Based on the daily requirements of the job, students can determine the steps to take to make positive physical and behavioral changes. For example, changes could include modifying the frequency, intensity, duration, and types of exercise activities to maximize the benefits of routine exercise, and reducing health issues related to inactivity and the potential for injury.

Basics of Goal Setting

Goal setting is a simple but often overlooked behavioral skill that provides you with a sense of order and control in stressful situations. Knowingly and deliberately setting goals allows you to set a direction. Regular evaluation of your goals and objectives helps you to mark progress and make adjustments as necessary. This tool provides you with some degree of control over individual stressors. Setting goals helps you organize your stressors and your responses to them, ideally one stressor at a time.

How do you set a goal? Initially, consider the goal to be what you wish to accomplish. The goal needs to be realistically attainable and measurable. Goals should be written in a manner that allows you to measure their progress and completion; this includes identifying the steps necessary to meet the goal so that when all the steps are completed the goal will be satisfied. It is okay to develop as many steps as needed to identify key processes in attaining the goal and to mark progress. As each step is completed, it is checked off.

For example, you set for yourself the goal of recognizing the effect of stress on your eating habits. The steps might be to recognize stressors and determine their relationship to what is eaten, when, and how much. This presumes that you have already recognized that you are experiencing stress and that you think it is having an impact on your eating habits because your clothes have become either too tight or too loose.

Setting goals and achieving them can help to make work, stress, and life more manageable. Proven methods that make goal setting a productive and positive experience include the following six key components:

- **Set clear, specific goals.** Make them as detailed as possible, because the details will allow you to plan for potential roadblocks that could arise along the way.

- **Take small steps.** Accomplish short-term goals on the path to your long-term goal. Take time to celebrate each success!
- **Get support.** This should be helpful and honest support to provide you the most help. Support can be professional or social.
- **Share your goals with others.** Sharing will help you maintain accountability in achieving success.
- **Stay positive.** Maintain optimism when roadblocks appear, because they tend to be temporary. Reach out to your support network as they can help motivate you to keep going.
- **Track successes and challenges.** Be prepared to transition or modify your path along the way. Writing down your successes and challenges will prove that you are moving forward.

Cognitive Skills and Cognitive Therapy Skills

The cognitive skills of perspective, understanding self-defeating thoughts, empathy, and dealing with wins and losses allow EMS practitioners to mentally cope with stress. In the simplest sense, you might view your interaction with the world as a series of events that lead to consequences or outcomes. Although you cannot control what life throws your way, you can control your reactions to life's events. You can begin by identifying those beliefs that erode your ability to effectively deal with stress and constructing beliefs that better allow you to deal with stress. These more robust and positive beliefs allow you to better put things into perspective and improve your critical thinking skills in difficult situations, and they provide you with better strategies for how to deal with the wins and losses associated with EMS and life in general.

Some might say that cognitive skills are best developed through working with a therapist. In addition, there are numerous books, websites, and apps that can teach you relaxation and meditation skills. The following skills can help EMS practitioners to cope with stress:

- **Progressive relaxation and controlled breathing.** This practice enables you to calm your mind, decrease anxiety, and gain perspective about your beliefs. Effective relaxation techniques can provide a healthy approach to working through stressful calls/situations that you have encountered.
- **Cognitive restructuring.** A process that encourages people to address their negative thinking patterns. It helps you to view a situation in the right context, helps with empathy and sympathy, and understand self-defeating thoughts.

- **Assertiveness training.** This allows you to have difficult conversations with yourself and others.
- **Problem-solving techniques.** These can help you plan your recovery to cope with wins and losses.

Building Social Skills

Because EMS practitioners are those to whom people in great need reach for help, it can be uncomfortable for EMS practitioners to reach out to others for help. Among EMS practitioners, there is significant stigma attached to reaching out. The Code Green Campaign is just one organization that is actively working to reduce that stigma. A social network is a safety net for stressful, complex situations. This group is defined in your goal setting. That is, when you set goals, identify who in your social network can help support you as you try to achieve your goals. Know the roles of each person in your group. Know who are the empathetic listeners, who will always tell you the truth and not just what you want to hear, and who you can call at any hour to talk.

How do you go about developing a social support system? Identify the personal characteristics that you look for in people in your support system. Identify the people you want in your support system and, importantly, identify the role each person plays in your support system.

Next, identify the personal characteristics that you provide to your social support system. Identify your strengths and weaknesses. The process of identifying your strengths can help you to become more self-efficacious. **Self-efficacy** is the belief that you are capable of performing in a certain way to achieve a certain goal. For example, if an EMS practitioner was able to remain committed to a diet and exercise program, even during extended weight loss plateaus, he or she could recall that same discipline and self-belief and apply it when facing a new life challenge.

Stay in the Field

Organizations that have resources designed to help deal with stress include the following:

- The Code Green Campaign
- American Psychological Association's Road to Resilience
- American Foundation for Suicide Prevention
- American Association of Suicidology
- International Association for Suicide Prevention
- National Suicide Prevention Lifeline (1-800-273-8255)

Finally, identify the actions that you might use to improve your support system. Always remember that the social support process is very much a two-way street. Consider what *you* can give back to your support system. Also remember that it is far easier to develop a social support system before a crisis occurs.

Resilience can act as a buffer against developing PTSD. The average lifetime risk for developing PTSD is 3.5% in the general public and 34% in EMS. Resilience can also assist in developing **posttraumatic growth (PTG)**. PTG is an emerging field of study that demonstrates that survivors of trauma can actually grow and become "better people" through their willingness to build greater resilience skills from the traumas they have confronted. Resilience skills can empower people to become better caregivers to our patients, families, communities, and, ultimately, ourselves.

Stay in the Field

Therapeutic techniques that have been developed to help people process trauma and unpleasant life events, which may be employed by trained therapists, include the following:

- **Eye movement desensitization reprocessing (EMDR) therapy.** This therapy has been proven to help people with anxiety, depression, and PTSD. Treatment focuses on changing thoughts, emotions, or behaviors through targeting:
  - The memories of the events that are linked to the emotional, cognitive, and behavioral problems.
  - Conditions that could trigger a dysfunction.
  - Incorporating skill to address future occurrences.
- **Emotional freedom technique (EFT).** This is a self-help therapeutic technique associated with tapping acupoints while repeating a phrase of how you feel. This technique has been heavily researched, and one study supported a 90% improvement score compared to 63% from those receiving cognitive behavioral therapy.

CHAPTER WRAP-UP

- Add physical fitness into daily routines.
- Eating and hydrating well requires planning, preparation, and making good choices.
- Sleep is the only way to reduce sleep debt.
- Understand fatigue countermeasures.
- Proactively identify stressors.
- Develop stress management practices, such as resilience skills.

SUMMARY

- Mental health impacts relationships, decision-making abilities, and the ability to handle stress.
- Stress is any event or situation that creates not only an emotional response but also physical and psychological responses. When stress occurs, the person can perceive the event as harmful, threatening, or challenging.

- Eustress is positive, beneficial short-term stress. With eustress, psychological balance is restored when a person sees that he or she is capable of tackling life's happier challenges, such as getting married or buying a home.
- Distress disrupts a person's psychological balance and can overwhelm him or her physically and

(continued)

SUMMARY (continued)

mentally. Distress includes losing a family member or experiencing a serious illness or injury.

- The day-to-day stressors experienced in the EMS workplace include handling changing work schedules and enduring rudeness from others.

- Depression occurs when a person loses interest or pleasure in living. A person with depression may lose the ability to concentrate, which makes it more difficult to take an interest in the activities of daily life.

- Anxiety is a vague feeling of dread. Physical, emotional, mental, and behavioral reactions can occur simultaneously. Procrastination and social isolation can occur in people with anxiety.

- Long-term stressors inherent in EMS include a low and/or unpredictable income.

- Sleep and relaxation are important assets in the resilience toolbox, because exhaustion is a major component of burnout.

- Sleep debt is the difference between the amount of sleep you get and the amount that your body needs. Unfortunately, you cannot pay back the sleep debt in a lump sum. Sleep debts impact your behavior and can negatively impact you both physically and mentally.

- Physical fitness is a requirement of being an EMS practitioner. An EMS practitioner must be able to bend, twist, reach, and pull repetitively in a manner that hurts neither the EMS practitioner nor the patient. As an EMS practitioner, you need to have functional strength, stability, and mobility to tolerate the stresses imposed on your body on a daily basis.

- Fitness is a critical component of overall physical and mental wellness, in addition to being able to meet the physical requirements of the job. Regular physical activity, healthy eating, and stress reduction all improve overall wellness.

- Resilience skills enable people to adapt and manage both daily stressors and major life events.

- The first skills in the resilience toolbox are the physical and behavioral skills that help provide optimal physical health. The skills are goal setting, healthy eating, exercise, sleep, relaxation, and building social skills.

GLOSSARY

anxiety A vague feeling of dread accompanied by activation of the autonomic nervous system to produce both physical and mental sensations ranging from dizziness to panic.

depression A mood disorder characterized by persistent feelings of sadness.

distress A disruption of a person's psychological balance that can produce extreme anxiety, sorrow, or pain.

eustress Short-term stress that is positive and beneficial; psychological balance is restored when a person sees that he or she is capable of tackling life's happy challenges.

microsleep When the mind ceases to be aware of its surroundings and the eyes may close for a short period; it may last from a few seconds to a few minutes.

post-traumatic growth (PTG) An emerging field of study that demonstrates that survivors of trauma can grow and make new meaning from traumas they have confronted.

resilience The ability to cope with stress and adversity without suffering lasting physical or psychological harm.

self-efficacy The belief that you are capable of performing in a certain way to achieve a certain goal.

sleep debt The difference between the amount of sleep you get and the amount that your body needs.

stress Physical, chemical, or emotional factors that cause positive negative physical or psychological tension.

REFERENCES

Abbott C, Barber E, Burke BA, et al. What's Killing our Medics? Reviving Responders: Ambulance Service Manager Program. Published April 21, 2015. Accessed March 30, 2021. https://static1.squarespace.com/static/555d1154e4b09b430c18fd39/t/5599d2b2e4b0c805c287aa3a/1436144306212/What%27s+Killing+Our+Medics+Final.pdf

About The Code Green Campaign. The Code Green Campaign. Published 2021. Accessed May 18, 2021. https://codegreencampaign.org/.

American College of Cardiology. Physical Activity Guidelines for Americans. Published November 14, 2018. Accessed February 4, 2021. https://www.acc.org/latest-in-cardiology/ten-points-to-remember/2018/11/14/14/37/the-physical-activity-guidelines-for-americans

American Council on Exercise. *Task Performance and Health Improvement Recommendations for Emergency Medical Service Practitioners.* San Diego, CA: ACE; 2012.

American Foundation for Suicide Prevention. Suicide statistics. Published 2021. Accessed December 17, 2021. https://afsp.org/suicide-statistics/

Association for Behavioral and Cognitive Therapies. CBT Therapy for Stress. Published 2021. Accessed April 5, 2021. https://www.abct.org/Information/?m=mInformation&fa=fs_STRESS

Bach D, Groesbeck G, Stapleton P, Sims R, Blickheuser K, Church D. Clinical EFT (emotional freedom techniques) improves multiple physiological markers of health. *J Evid Based Integr Med.* 2019;24:2515690X18823691. doi:10.1177/2515690X18823691

Beaton R. Extreme stress: promoting resilience among EMS workers. *Northwest Pub Health.* 2006;23(2):8-9.

Benedict C, Cedernaes J, Giedraitis V, et al. Acute sleep deprivation and neurodegeneration. *Sleep.* 2014;37(1):195-198.

Boath E, Good R, Tsaroucha A, Stewart T, Pitch S, Boughey AJ. Tapping your way to success: using emotional freedom techniques (EFT) to reduce anxiety and improve communication skills in social work students. *Social Work Ed.* 2017;36(6):715-730. doi:10.1080/02615479.2017.1297394

Bohström D, Carlström E, Sjöström N. Managing stress in prehospital care: strategies used by ambulance nurses. *Int Emerg Nurs.* 2017;32:28-33. doi:10.1016/j.ienj.2016.08.004

Butkowski TJ. Sleepy and unfit. *Saf Health.* 2014;189(6):66-67.

Camart N, Sbeira F, Romo L. Can we learn to manage stress? A randomized controlled trial carried out on university students. van Wouwe JP, ed. *PLoS One.* 2018;13(9):e0200997. doi:10.1371/journal.pone.0200997

Centers for Disease Control and Prevention, National Center for Injury Prevention and Control. Web-based Injury Statistics Query and Reporting System (WISQARS) [online]. 2010.

Clarke SP, Oades LG, Crowe TP, Deane FP. Collaborative goal technology: theory and practice. *Psych Rehab J.* 2006;30(2):129-136. doi:10.2975/30.2006.129.136

Cook G. *Athletic Body in Balance.* Champagne, IL: Human Kinetics; 2003.

De Jongh A, Amann BL, Hofmann A, Farrell D, Lee CW. The status of EMDR therapy in the treatment of posttraumatic stress disorder 30 years after its introduction. *J EMDR Pract Res.* 13(4):261-269. doi:10.1891/1933-3196.13.4.261

Gavidia M. A rare gene mutation is associated with requiring less sleep, researchers say. *Am J Manag Care.* Published August 28, 2019. Accessed March 30, 2021. https://www.ajmc.com/view/a-rare-gene-mutation-is-associated-with-requiring-less-sleep-researchers-say

Gist R, Taylor VH, Raak S. White paper: suicide surveillance, prevention, and intervention measures for the US Fire Services. Presented at: The Suicide and Depression Summit July 11-12, 2011; Baltimore, MD: National Fallen Firefighters Foundation.

Gotlib I, Hammen C. *Handbook of Depression.* New York, NY: Guilford Press; 2002.

Gunderson J, Grill M, Callahan P, Marks M. Responder resilience. *JEMS.* 2014;39(3):57-61.

Hase M. The structure of EMDR therapy: a guide for the therapist. *Front Psychol.* 2021;12. doi:10.3389/fpsyg.2021.660753

Kilbourne AM, Beck K, Spaeth-Rublee B, et al. Measuring and improving the quality of mental health care: a global perspective. *World Psych.* 2018;17(1):30-38. doi:10.1002/wps.20482

Kirkwood C. Tricking taste buds but not the brain: artificial sweeteners change brain. Scientific American, MIND Guest Blog. September 5, 2013. Accessed December 8, 2021. https://blogs.scientificamerican.com/mind-guest-blog/tricking-taste-buds-but-not-the-brain-artificial-sweeteners-change-braine28099s-pleasure-response-to-sweet/

Lehmann C. Slow waves of CSF during sleep clear toxins linked to neurodegenerative conditions. *Neurol Today.* 2019;19(23):9-10. doi:10.1097/01.nt.0000617164.64963.90

Leiter MP, Maslach C. Conquering burnout. *Sci American Mind.* 2015;26(1):30-35.

Maguire BJ, Hunting KL, Smith GS, Levick NR. Occupational fatalities in emergency medical services: a hidden crisis. *Ann Emer Med.* 2002;40:625-632.

Maguire BJ, Smith S. Injuries and fatalities among emergency medical technicians in the United States. *Prehosp Disaster Med.* 2013;28(4):376-382.

Mental Health America. Work Life Balance. Published 2021. Accessed February 1, 2021. https://www.mhanational.org/work-life-balance

Mountfort S, Wilson J. EMS Provider Health and Wellness. StatPearls [Internet]. Last revised September 28, 2021. Accessed March 30, 2021. https://www.ncbi.nlm.nih.gov/books/NBK493236/

Murray CJL, Lopez AD, eds. *The Global Burden of Disease: A Comprehensive Assessment of Mortality and Morbidity from Diseases, Injuries and Risk Factors in 1990 and Projected to 2020.* Cambridge, MA: Harvard University Press; 1996.

National Association of Emergency Medical Technicians. Guide to Building an Effective EMS Wellness and Resilience Program. Published 2019. Accessed March 31, 2021. http://www.naemt.org/docs/default-source/ems-preparedness/naemt-resilience-guide-01-15-2019-final.pdf?Status=Temp&sfvrsn=d1edc892_2

National Institutes of Health. How Sleep Clears the Brain. Published October 28, 2013. Accessed February 4, 2021.

https://www.nih.gov/news-events/nih-research-matters/how-sleep-clears-brain

Nedergaard M. Garbage truck of the brain. *Science.* 2013;340(28):1529-1530.

Patterson PD, Weaver MD, Frank RC, et al. Association between poor sleep, fatigue, and safety outcomes in emergency medical services providers. *Prehosp Emerg Care.* 2012;16(1):86-97. doi:10.3109/10903127.2011.616261

Randall CL, McNeil DW. Motivational interviewing as an adjunct to cognitive behavior therapy for anxiety disorders: a critical review of the literature. *Cogn Behav Pract.* 2017;24(3):296-311. doi:10.1016/j.cbpra.2016.05.003

Rothbaum B. *Pathological Anxiety: Emotional Processing in Etiology and Treatment.* New York, NY: Guilford Press; 2006.

Russo MB, Kendall AP, Johnson DE, et al. Visual perception, psychomotor performance, and complex motor performance during an overnight air refueling simulated flight. *Aviat Space Environ Med.* 2005;76(7 Suppl):C92-C103.

Saleh D, Seaward BL. *Managing Stress: Principles and Strategies for Health and Well Being.* Burlington, MA: Jones & Bartlett Learning; 2018.

Shapiro F, Wesselmann D, Mevissen L. Eye movement desensitization and reprocessing therapy (EMDR). In: Landolt M, Cloitre M, Schnyder U (eds). *Evidence-Based Treatments for Trauma*

Related Disorders in Children and Adolescents. Springer, Cham; 2017. doi:10.1007/978-3-319-46138-0_13

Shi G, Xing L, Wu D, et al. A rare mutation of β1-adrenergic receptor affects sleep/wake behaviors. *Neuron.* 2019;103(6):1044-1055.e7. doi:10.1016/j.neuron.2019.07.026

Suni E. How much sleep do we really need? The Sleep Foundation. Updated March 10, 2021. Accessed October 20, 2021. https://www.sleepfoundation.org/how-sleep-works/how-much-sleep-do-we-really-need/page/0,1

The American Institute of Stress. What is Stress? Published 2011. Updated 2020. Accessed February 1, 2021. https://www.stress.org/daily-life

Tsismenakis AJ, Christophi CA, Burress JW, Kinney AM, Kim M, Kales SN. The obesity epidemic and future emergency responders. *Obesity.* 2009;17(8):1648-1650.

U.S. Department of Agriculture. MyPlate. Published 2021. Accessed February 4, 2021. https://www.myplate.gov

Valtin H. "Drink at least eight glasses of water a day." Really? Is there scientific evidence for "8 × 8"? *Am J Physiol Regul Integr Comp Physiol.* 2002;283(5):R993-R1004. doi:10.1152/ajpregu.00365.2002

Wehrenberg M, Prinz S. *The Anxious Brain.* New York, NY: W.W. Norton and Company; 2007.

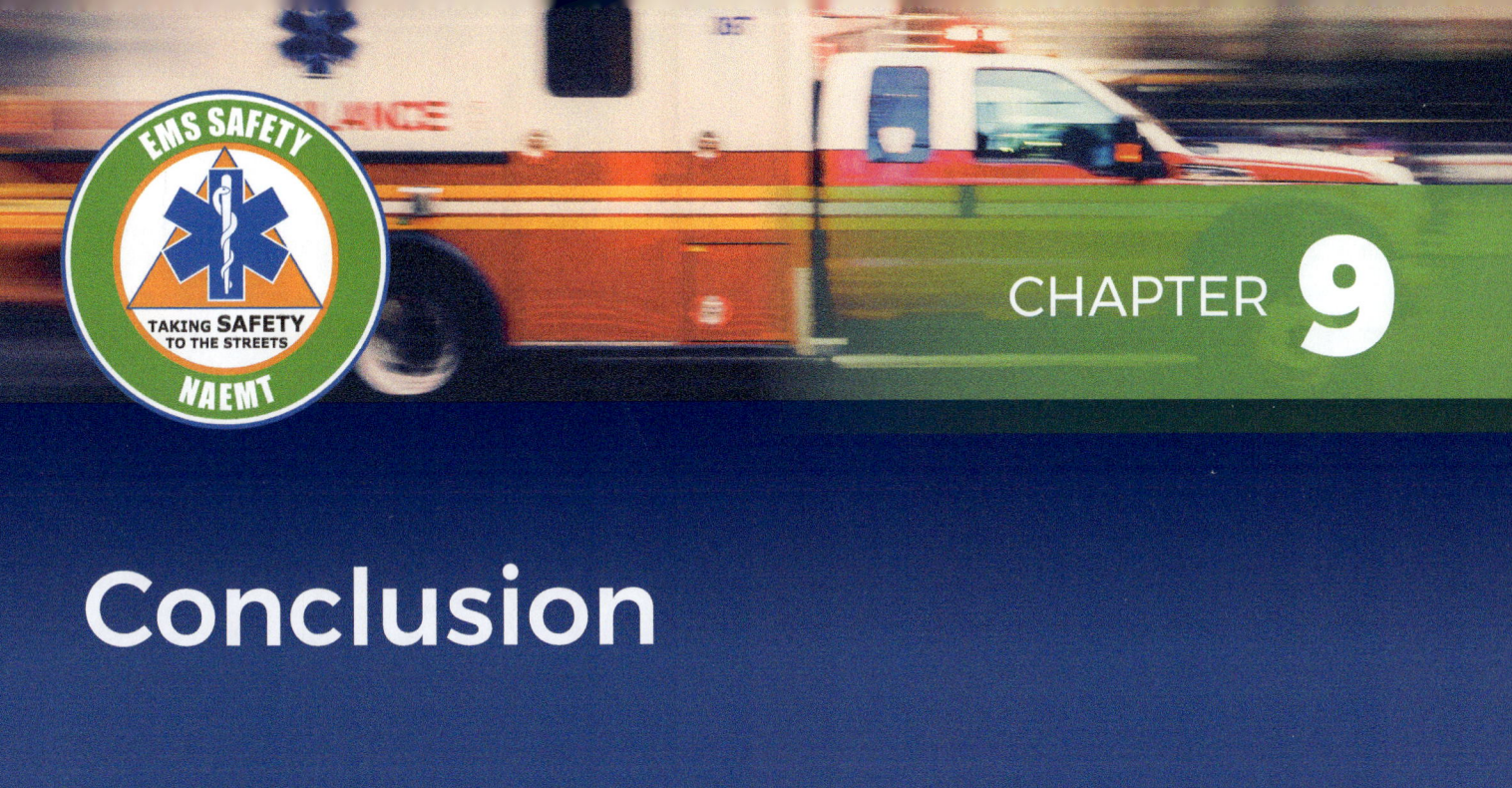

CHAPTER 9

Conclusion

Scenario

You and your partner have had a busy shift and are returning to quarters. You are driving in moderate traffic and discussing after-work plans when your cell phone rings. Glancing down at the phone, you see that it's your spouse calling. As you reach down to pick up the phone, you hear your partner exclaim, "Red light, red light, RED LIGHT!" Halfway through the intersection you hear metal on metal when a vehicle hits your ambulance on the passenger side. Your ambulance rolls over and is pushed across the intersection, coming to a sudden stop after striking a telephone pole. When the airbags deflate, you look over to see your partner unconscious, bleeding from the head, while you are dangling upside down, held in place by your seat belt.

1. What is your first responsibility when driving an ambulance?
2. How should this type of distraction be handled?
3. What is your next action?

Introduction

How you behave on every call impacts your safety, your patients' safety, and the safety of the community at large (**FIGURE 9-1**). If you drive too fast for the current road conditions, you put all of the ambulance occupants and the general public at risk of injury. If you don't buckle your seat belt before the ambulance starts moving, your patients will notice. Such behaviors are observed and assessed by the public. When members of the public see emergency medical services (EMS) practitioners engaging in unsafe behaviors, they may deem it appropriate to engage in the same unsafe behaviors. The status of the overtly unsafe EMS practitioner may

diminish the profession in the eyes of the public, who may be less likely to follow instructions from caregivers they do not respect.

In addition to modeling safe behaviors, you must create an environment in which respect among your colleagues is a given. Good communication will not occur without respect. Lapses in communication may prevent vital information from being shared. For further discussion, see Chapter 2, *Crew Resource Management*. The chain of survival applies to each of us; if one of us is unsafe, all of us are unsafe.

As an EMS practitioner, you must be active, educated, and well practiced regarding all facets of safety. When it comes to safety, there is no room for an attitude

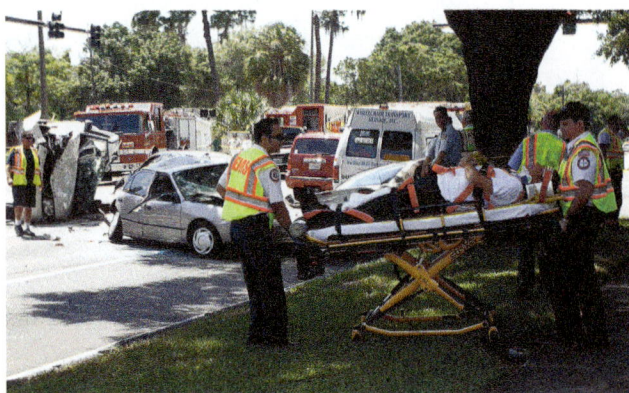

FIGURE 9-1 How you behave on every call impacts your safety, your patients' safety, and the safety of the community at large.

© St. Petersburg Times/ZUMApress.com/Alamy Stock Photo.

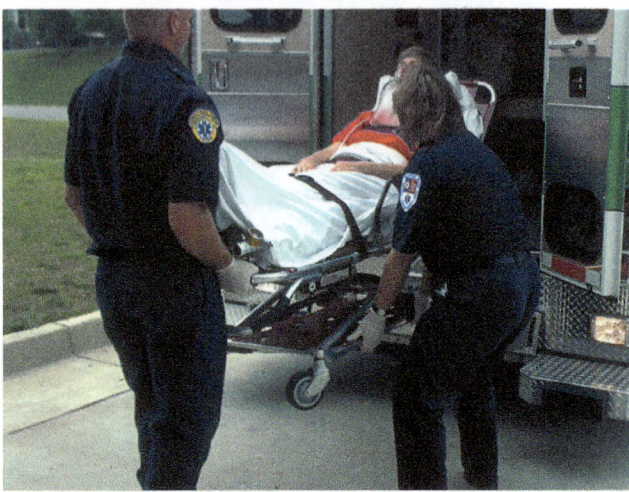

FIGURE 9-2 The ambulance is your mobile office.

© Jones & Bartlett Learning. Courtesy of MIEMSS.

In the Field

Good management practices must be embraced by those who develop them and by those who perform them on a daily basis. In addition, adequate resources must be supplied for the workforce to function safely. Finally, the workforce must adhere to safety policies and use the resources supplied by management.

of "that's not my job." In addition to having the skills obtained from mandatory safety training, you must be perceptive, recognize new hazards, and actively engage in mitigating those hazards.

As an EMS practitioner, you must be open to change and constructive criticism. Shared ignorance benefits nobody. Join professional organizations and participate in their activities. Subscribe to professional journals to enhance your awareness of what other EMS professionals experience.

Engage in dialogue with other professionals, not just those in EMS. Do you think that public health officials, infectious disease specialists, design engineers, or risk managers/engineers may have information from which you could benefit? You cannot limit the scope of your perspective to EMS. Other medical professionals have access to information that is not EMS specific but is vital for you to know. The risks from new infectious diseases or the enhanced risks from old ones are first recognized in the public health and infectious disease arenas, often well in advance of their emergence as EMS concerns. Engineers have knowledge that can affirm or refute the practicality of ideas that EMS practitioners have regarding ambulance design.

Significant Steps in Creating an EMS Culture of Safety

Ambulance

The ambulance is your place of business (**FIGURE 9-2**). As such, it must be designed in such a fashion that it can be used safely. This is such a critical issue that organizations such as the Commission for the Accreditation of Ambulance Services (CAAS), the National Fire Protection Association (NFPA), and the U.S. General Services Administration (GSA) have developed design standards for ground ambulances, which include the Ground Vehicle Standard for Ambulances (GVS V2.0), NFPA 1917: Standard for Automotive Ambulances, and KKK-A-1822F, respectively. It is wise to familiarize yourself with the most recent version of these standards, including any change notices, because different agencies will follow a specific standard based on their affiliation.

The intended performance of the ambulance is the basis for the design standards. The design standards factor in the environmental conditions in which the vehicle will be used, such as weather and terrain. The external structure is designed to protect occupants from the impact of external forces. The roads and traffic flow are considered in determining the best mechanical design.

The internal structure of the ambulance should be free from sharp edges, protrusions, and any other hazards. The design of the patient care compartment should be based on the movements required for EMS practitioners to provide patient care. EMS practitioners should be able to reach both the equipment and the

In the Field

The concept that the ambulance is your office mirrors the idea that EMS is a business. In some cases, it is a business in which profit is not a goal. However, the cost of operations is a critical component that must be evaluated for the survivability of any EMS system. How much does it cost to run and maintain an ambulance for an average transport? What is the ambulance's replacement cost? The agency's managers must apply the same level of intensity to fiscal efficiency as EMS practitioners do to clinical efficiency in the field.

patient while wearing proper restraints. This promotes operational efficiency as well as safety.

The driver and all ambulance occupants must have restraint systems that have been proven to safely secure them and a solid structure in the ambulance to absorb potential traumatic forces. Design engineers consider the worst-case scenarios, such as rollovers and high-speed crashes, when creating the structural and restraint system designs.

An interdisciplinary approach to ambulance design brings engineers, manufacturers, salespeople, purchasers, and EMS practitioners together. Technological advances in multiple arenas occur concurrently, so keeping information in professional silos is unproductive. For example, unless a design engineer receives input from an EMS practitioner, how will the design engineer know how large to make a space for the securement of a defibrillator?

Stay in the Field

Just as emerging technologies partially shape the standards of care, nonclinical technologies partially shape the standards of safety. Computer-aided dispatch, global positioning systems (GPS), and onboard monitoring systems continue to advance in complexity and effectiveness. However, you must understand that no technology is a panacea. It must be used in a thoughtful and systematic manner.

NAEMT

The National Association of Emergency Medical Technicians (NAEMT) EMS Workforce Committee influences the operational standards of EMS systems through the development of professional standards for EMS in position papers. NAEMT position papers demonstrate the unity of the goals within the EMS community as a whole and the needs of EMS practitioners. The acquisition of resources by EMS systems for the protection and safety of EMS practitioners is more likely to occur when the importance of safety is called out as a common goal for the EMS profession to achieve.

NAEMT also expresses the importance of safety through the development of continuing education courses, such as EMS Safety and Emergency Vehicle Operator Safety (EVOS), which were developed to address the unacceptable levels of death, injury, and illness seen among EMS practitioners.

Federal Regulations

The awareness of the dangers to which EMS practitioners and all first responders are exposed when responding to emergencies on highways led to federal legislation requiring emergency responders to wear high-visibility safety vests. Although the legislation on the wearing of these vests focused on federal highways, the federal government's emphasis on the importance of safety vests as a key tool in preventing injury and deaths in first responders resulted in their use becoming commonplace on all roadways. Remember, "When your feet are on the street, the vest is on your chest."

The National Highway Traffic Safety Administration's (NHTSA) Office of EMS has a webpage on safety that is focused on "protecting the health and safety of EMS practitioners and their patients." This page offers viewers links to NHTSA projects on topics such as fatigue in EMS, provider and patient safety, webinars on reducing workforce injuries or reducing opioid overdoses, and articles on preventing injuries and other safety topics.

Stay in the Field

Safe EMS practitioners have longer and more comfortable careers. It is easier to function and stick around if you are healthy and uninjured!

EMS Culture of Safety

Safety Begins With You

You will not be safe unless you come to work mentally and physically prepared every day. This takes planning, preparation, and discipline. Without a "sound mind in a healthy body," you will not be able to effectively

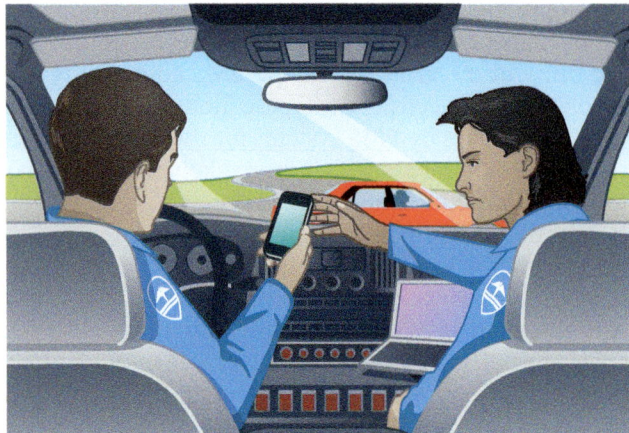

FIGURE 9-3 If you see a potential hazard, speak up! Warn others and take action to eliminate the hazard.

© Jones & Bartlett Learning.

process the information in your work environment. You will not recognize the potential dangers. What you do not recognize, you cannot share. This places you and your coworkers in harm's way.

In the Field

Share what you have learned in this text. You do not have to give a formal lecture; you can instruct your coworkers through your safety-conscious behaviors. Don't just talk the talk; be sure to walk the walk as a role model!

Do not engage in unsafe behaviors, and do not tolerate them in others. When you see hazards, act (**FIGURE 9-3**). Immediately communicate the presence of the potential hazards to anyone in the area who may be harmed. Take immediate action to minimize the impact of the unsafe conditions, and inform your management team as necessary.

Do not get lulled into a false sense of security. Analyze your behaviors and those of your coworkers, not just individually but collectively. Talk with your peers and think out loud with each other. It can be as simple as, "We should have moved the table before we moved the patient." Or it could be, "We need new wiper blades right now. Call dispatch."

Stay in the Field

Emergency vehicle operators should always drive the ambulance safely, without distraction, and ambulance crew members should require anyone who drives them to behave in the same manner.

In the Field

What are some things you can do today, tomorrow, next week, and next month to keep building the EMS culture of safety?

- **Talk the talk.** Talk to others in your EMS system about what you have learned and how it can apply to them and the EMS system.
- **Walk the walk (or drive the ambulance).**
  - Use what you have learned to lead by example. Be a safe EMS practitioner.
  - Get some sleep!
  - Put your cell phone away.
- **Lead the charge.**
  - Talk with your superiors and let them know the benefits of creating a safer work environment and the dangers of *not* doing so.
  - Participate in near-miss (close calls) and crash reviews.
  - Join your EMS system's safety committee.
- **Keep up to date.**
  - Use the *EMS Safety* text as a reference for the future.
  - Read the increasing number of articles on EMS safety topics in the major EMS and fire service magazines.
  - Join an online EMS safety discussion group.
  - Sign up for alerts from NHTSA, *EMS World*, EMS1, the Occupational Safety and Health Administration (OSHA), and the Centers for Disease Control and Prevention (CDC).
  - Continue your NAEMT membership (when you take the EMS Safety course, you will receive a free 1-year introductory membership).
- **Be open to new ideas.**
  - Major design changes may be proposed in vehicles and equipment. Evaluate the changes objectively and be an advocate for those changes that will benefit you and your EMS system.
  - Think of ways to make your workplace safer and submit ideas to your supervisors; do not just talk about them.
- **Become an NAEMT instructor for *EMS Safety*.** This will enable you to share the information you have learned with your EMS system and other EMS agencies in your region.

Promote formal reporting processes. Incident reports can be used to identify hazards, quantify them, and monitor trends. Near-miss reporting, or the recognition of hazardous events that almost happened but did not, helps to identify results based on simple luck as compared with those based on good preventive practices. Near-miss reports can provide crucial insights that can be used to develop safety practice standards. If your EMS system has a safety committee, be an active member on it, or at least provide input to the committee.

Continuous learning will keep your mind open to new ideas. Open-mindedness will allow you to evaluate new ideas objectively. Use critical reasoning when presented with proposed design changes in vehicles and equipment. Do not reject or accept anything solely on the basis that it is new.

Constantly think about ways to make your workplace safer, share your ideas with your coworkers, and submit them to management. When it comes to safety, do not forget that little things matter, too. Do you need more lighting in the garage? Are the steps slick? Does the station keep running out of hand sanitizer in the bathroom?

Wrap-Up

How can you best wrap up this *EMS Safety* text and the EMS Safety course? We suggest you now review each of the "wrap-ups" listed here and make them your action plan as you begin to develop a culture of safety in your organization!

CHAPTER WRAP-UPS

Chapter 1: How Safety Impacts Patients and Practitioners
- The goal of EMS Safety is to create a culture of safety in EMS.
- Self-injury prevention is the most valuable service a prehospital provider can provide.
- Everyone is responsible for the commitment to fostering a culture of safety.
- Effective communication and documentation are critical components to implementing a culture of safety.

Chapter 2: Crew Resource Management
- CRM helps reduce the inherent risk of EMS.
- CRM cannot guarantee absolute safety.
- CRM is only one of many tools that organizations can use to manage errors.

Chapter 3: Emergency Vehicle Safety
- Respect your vehicle and safety equipment.
- When operating emergency vehicles drive with due regard using defensive driving techniques.
- Avoid common emergency vehicle accidents.
- Use caution while driving emergently.
- Be mindful of patient compartment risks.

Chapter 4: Safety in the Roadway
- Roadway operations are a real safety threat.
- Traffic incident management plans are critical to reduce injuries and fatalities.
- Wear a high-visibility safety vest day and night.
- Use the appropriate number of lights with the right lighting during roadway operations.
- Communicate with air medical services to ensure safety for all.

Chapter 5: Patient Safety
- Making patient safety a high priority should be a goal for all providers.
- Identify barriers in patient safety and the steps to improve them.
- Near-misses are warning signs that should be taken seriously.
- Just culture aims to create an environment in which people feel empowered to report errors and adverse events.
- Complacency is dangerous and unacceptable.

(continued)

CHAPTER WRAP-UPS (continued)

Chapter 6: Practitioner Safety From Violence
- Every scene has the potential for violence.
- Situational awareness on all scenes is critical.
- Use nonverbal and verbal communication techniques for de-escalation.
- If restraints—physical and/or pharmacologic—are required, ensure patient and responder safety.
- Above all, your safety is most important!

Chapter 7: Injury and Infection Prevention
- Injury prevention begins prior to the shift.
- Use lift assist teams when available.
- Prepare the patient compartment so that seat belts can be used by providers.
- Utilize proper PPE based on the pathogen of concern.
- Don and doff PPE properly.
- Provide masks to patients to ensure source control.

Chapter 8: Personal Health
- Add physical fitness into daily routines.
- Eating and hydrating well requires planning, preparation, and making good choices.
- Sleep is the only way to reduce sleep debt.
- Understand fatigue countermeasures.
- Proactively identify stressors.
- Develop stress management practices, such as resilience skills.

SUMMARY

- How you behave on every call impacts your safety, your patients' safety, and the safety of the community at large.

- When members of the public see EMS practitioners engaging in unsafe behaviors, they may deem it appropriate to engage in the same unsafe behaviors.

- Safety depends on good communication. Good communication occurs in an environment where everyone is respected.

- As EMS practitioners, you must be active, educated, and well practiced in all facets of safety. In addition to the skills obtained from mandatory safety training, you must recognize new hazards and actively engage in mitigating them.

- As EMS practitioners, you must be open to change and constructive criticism. You can enhance your awareness of what other EMS professionals experience by joining professional organizations, subscribing to professional journals, and speaking with a diverse range of professionals, from public health workers to ambulance engineers.

- NAEMT influences safety in EMS through the development of professional standards for EMS in position papers and through the development of continuing education courses, such as EMS Safety.

- Do not engage in unsafe behaviors, and do not tolerate them in others. When you see hazards, act.

- Do not get lulled into a false sense of security. Analyze your behaviors and those of your coworkers, not just individually but collectively.

- Incident reports can be used to identify hazards, quantify them, and monitor trends. Near-miss reports can provide crucial insights that can be used to develop safety practice standards.

- Continuous learning keeps your mind open to new ideas. Open-mindedness allows you to evaluate new ideas objectively.

- All EMS practitioners should constantly think about ways to make their workplaces safer. Ideas should be shared with coworkers and submitted to management. Safety is both an individual and group effort.

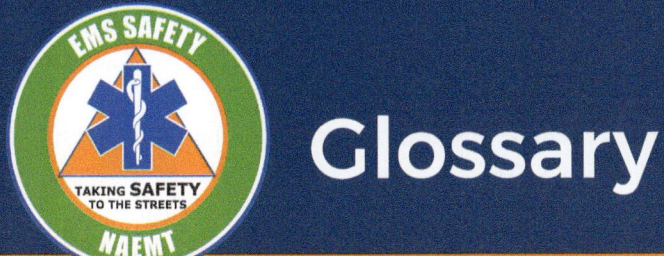

Glossary

adverse event: An event that results in harm to a patient.

aggressive driving: Operating a vehicle with aggressive actions, without concern for other drivers.

anxiety: A vague feeling of dread accompanied by activation of the autonomic nervous system to produce both physical and mental sensations ranging from dizziness to panic.

assessment "L" formation: A formation that permits one EMS practitioner to address the patient from the front and another EMS practitioner to remain at the patient's side, performing patient care. If the patient attacks, this formation provides the second EMS practitioner enough time to escape and call for help.

cachectic: Possessing an appearance of wasting away.

challenge: More direct than an alert; when a team member physically moves into the action circle, prepared to take the next step of emergency intervention.

cognitive distractions: Distractions that take the emergency vehicle operator's mind off the road and operation of the vehicle.

coherence: When a message is understood by the receiver.

complacency: A feeling of satisfaction with one's own performance to the point of not recognizing the potential for errors.

concealment: An object that hides a person from view but does not protect him or her from projectiles or a potential attacker.

conflict resolution: A range of processes aimed at alleviating or eliminating sources of conflict; generally includes negotiation, mediation, and diplomacy.

conspicuity: The ability of a vehicle to draw the attention of other drivers.

cover: A barrier that both hides and protects—for example, a brick wall, large rocks, or a vehicle engine block.

crew resource management (CRM): A tool originally instituted by the airline industry in 1980 to optimize performance and outcomes by reducing the effect of human error through the use of all available resources.

defensive stance: A position that creates a nonthreatening, nonaggressive appearance. The EMS practitioner stands with hands up and palms forward in an open position, keeping the elbows in and angling the body 45 degrees to the patient.

delirium with agitated behavior: A condition in which patients have an increased sympathetic response and may become agitated, violent, combative, or paranoid.

depression: A mood disorder characterized by persistent feelings of sadness.

direct costs: Those costs commonly associated with out-of-pocket payments. They include payments to physicians, rehabilitation professionals, insurance carriers, and attorneys.

distress: A disruption of a person's psychological balance that can produce extreme anxiety, sorrow, or pain.

due regard: The ethical, and sometimes legal, principle that guides vehicle operators to ensure overall safety to the general public, including actions needed to prevent the possibility of collision or unsafe behavior.

engineering controls: Changes made to the work environment through the use of equipment to avoid work-related injury (e.g., specialty stretchers, lateral transfer aids).

eustress: Short-term stress that is positive and beneficial; psychological balance is restored when a person sees that he or she is capable of tackling life's happy challenges.

hardware: Solutions that take the form of computers, vehicles, tools, medications, or protective equipment.

high-reliability organizations (HROs): Organizations that operate in high-risk environments yet strive to maintain a learning atmosphere so as to minimize chances for error.

human perception time: The rate at which a person perceives incoming stimuli.

human reaction time: The time it takes for a person to react to an impending event.

humanware: The people who are part of a team that has been directed to solve a particular problem.

indirect costs: Costs related to injury that are not covered by insurance. For example, lost productivity.

lift assist team: A team utilized to help EMS practitioners with patient lifting, it can be made up of additional responders on the scene, hospital staff, or another ambulance crew called in as backup.

manual distractions: Distractions that cause the emergency vehicle operator to take a hand off the ambulance steering wheel.

microsleep: When the mind ceases to be aware of its surroundings and the eyes may close for a short period; it may last from a few seconds to a few minutes.

near-miss event: An error in patient care that occurs but is caught before it reaches the patient.

no-harm event: An error in patient care that does not result in harm.

pharmacologic sedation: The use of medications to manage an agitated, combative, or violent patient to prevent self-harm.

post-incident analysis (PIA): An activity involving team members that takes place after an incident response. It reviews performance of individuals and teams while focusing on learning lessons that can be applied to future incidents.

post-traumatic growth (PTG): An emerging field of study that demonstrates that survivors of trauma can grow and make new meaning from traumas they have confronted.

proprioception: The reception and processing of sensory information that allows an individual to have an awareness of body position.

rate of closure: The speed at which one vehicle overtakes another.

resilience: The ability to cope with stress and adversity without suffering lasting physical or psychological harm.

safe patient movement behaviors: These behaviors involve movement actions selected by the EMS practitioner that minimize the risk of injury to patients, practitioners, and bystanders during patient movement events.

second victim syndrome (SVS): When caregivers who commit an error in patient care feel significant mental, physical, and social impacts as a result of the error.

self-efficacy: The belief that you are capable of performing in a certain way to achieve a certain goal.

sensorimotor cues: Sights, sounds, and smells that create an awareness of environmental conditions; this awareness may prompt a behavioral response.

sentinel event: A subcategory of adverse events that causes death, permanent harm, or severe temporary harm.

situational awareness: The state of being aware of what is happening around you and recognizing the potential for threats to yourself or others.

sleep debt: The difference between the amount of sleep you get and the amount that your body needs.

software: Solutions that take the form of rewriting training materials or procedures or developing checklists or policies.

stress: Physical, chemical, or emotional factors that cause positive or negative physical or psychological tension.

surveying stance: The body posture to take when defusing a stressful patient encounter. The body is slightly at an angle, with hands above the waist and out of the pockets, arms neutral, and knees slightly bent with the weight on the balls of the feet.

tapering: A method to gradually direct traffic flow into an unaffected lane.

TeamSTEPPS®: A teamwork-based system that stands for Team Strategies and Tools to Enhance Performance and Patient Safety.

traffic incident management (TIM) plan: A pre-planning document created with the input of all emergency responding agencies to ensure that all agencies will work together to secure the scene, maintain scene safety, care for and safely extract patients from the scene, and clear the scene as efficiently and safely as possible.

unsafe actions: Actions that can lead to errors, injuries, death, or destruction.

vehicle braking time: The time it takes for the vehicle to stop.

vehicle reaction time: The time between when the brake pedal is applied and when the brakes start working.

visual distractions: Distractions that take the emergency vehicle operator's eyes off the road.

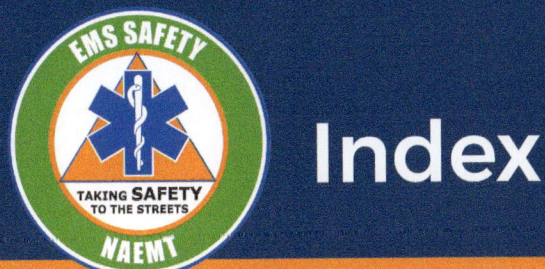

Index

Note: Page numbers followed by *f* and *t* denote figures and tables, respectively.